Menopause

Menopause

The Most Comprehensive,
Up-to-Date Information Available
to Help You Understand This Stage of Life,
Make the Right Treatment Choices,
and Cope Effectively

Isaac Schiff, M.D.
*Chief of Vincent Memorial
Obstetrics and Gynecology Service at
Massachusetts General Hospital*
with Ann B. Parson

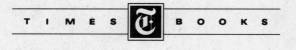

T I M E S 𝕿 B O O K S

R A N D O M   H O U S E

This book cannot and must not replace hands-on medical care or the specific advice of your doctor. Use it instead to help you ask the right questions, make the right choices, and work more closely with your doctor and other members of your health-care team.

Copyright © 1996 by The General Hospital Corporation

All rights reserved under International and Pan-American Copyright Conventions. Published in the United States by Times Books, a division of Random House, Inc., New York, and simultaneously in Canada by Random House of Canada Limited, Toronto.

Library of Congress Cataloging-in-Publication Data

Schiff, Isaac.
    Menopause: the most comprehensive, up-to-date information available to help you understand this stage of life, make the right treatment choices, and cope effectively / Isaac Schiff, with Ann B. Parson.—1st ed.
        p.   cm.
    Includes index.
    ISBN 0-8129-2318-9
    1. Menopause—Popular works.   2. Menopause—Hormone therapy.   I. Parson, Ann B.   II. Massachusetts General Hospital.
III. Title.
RG186.S35   1995
612.6'65—dc20   95-15171

Designed by Levavi & Levavi
Manufactured in the United States of America

9   8   7   6   5   4   3

To all my patients, who have given me the privilege of participating in their health care and whose insights keep teaching me and stimulating me to seek more knowledge

"Menopause came earlier than I expected—in my mid-forties. It really broke my heart because I always hoped to have children—the natural way. I'd always thought, Oh, there's plenty of time for that. Well, I ran out of time."

Acknowledgments

Several years ago, the staff of Massachusetts General Hospital set out to create a series of medical guides that would help all patients become more effective partners in their health care. We wanted to create clearly written, authoritative books that reflected a number of voices critical to the health care team, including doctors, nurses, dietitians, social workers, therapists, and, of course, the patients themselves.

Many people in many places have contributed to this guide to menopause. A great amount of appreciation is due all those concerned—the numerous researchers, nurses, staff members, and doctors who lent their time and expertise, and the numerous women who shared their experiences, making menopause and the years beyond that much more of an open book for other women.

For all their efforts, special thanks go to Martin Bander, Louise Braverman, Ruth Brown, Doe Coover, Sue Cummings, Madeline Drexler, Raja Sayegh, David Slovik, and Ann M. Voda. A wide circle of others also provided their knowledge and support. For their helpful involvement, appreciation goes to Nancy Avis, H. Leon Bradlow, Eugenia Calle, Karen J. Carlson, Mary Carey, Robin Cleary, Beverly Dammin, Cynthia D'Auria, Donald J. Deraska, Carolyn Develen, Maria A. Fiatarone, Marcha Flint, Rose Frisch, Henry Gewirtz, Annekathryn Goodman, Sherwood L. Gorbach, Diane Heislein, Tori Hudson, Elaine Kaye, Fredi Kronenberg, Barry I. Levine, Martha Marean, Elizabeth W. Markson, Kathy Martin, David T. MacLaughlin, Suzanne McGrail, John B. McKinlay, Irma L. Mebane-Sims, John E. Munzenrider, Robert M. Neer, Ann Nichols, George S. Richardson, Mary A. Riordan, Helen Strong, Wulf Utian, Dionysios Veronikis, Roberta Vitagliano, Judith Wurtman, and Ina Yalof.

Finally, thank you, Betsy Rapoport, for all your insight as editor.

Contents

Menopause

Introduction
Crossing the
Menopause Threshold

Not long ago, menopause was a subject surrounded by more silence than discussion, more myth than fact. In a few decades, however, science has raised our understanding of this transition point, clearing away misconceptions and promoting a new acceptance and awareness of menopause's biological intricacies.

Menopause isn't a disease, as earlier practitioners sometimes labeled it. Quite the opposite: It is a natural step in the process of aging. Just as menarche, the beginning of menstruation, signals the start of a woman's childbearing years, menopause signals the end of those years, and most women traverse it without serious medical or emotional complications. "I'm afraid I've begun menopause," one woman lamented to her physician. "Nonsense! You aren't going to pause for anything," the doctor objected. And that is true for the large majority of women. There's lots of life left beyond menopause; for most women, one-half of their adulthood. And contrary to the stereotypical view that life is all downhill after menopause, many women discover that the postmenopausal years offer fresh ground and bring new challenges.

Menopause's new visibility represents a valuable advance for women's health in this century. American female baby boomers—those born between 1946 and 1964—have been among the first to gain more control over their reproductive lives through advanced options in birth control, fertility, and abortion. Now, too, as they head toward menopause, they enjoy a new spectrum of health care choices. They have the advantage of knowing what to expect when menopause arrives and how to manage this passage, if they need to.

But perhaps most important, women today have the opportunity to use menopause as a yardstick for assessing their future health needs. Although the menopausal transition itself carries no health risks, a woman does encounter increased health risks after menopause, with the incidence rate for heart disease and osteoporosis (a thinning of bone) rising quite significantly. In the United States, health problems burden approximately 26 percent of women aged 65 and older. Older women, who live on average seven years longer than men, have more operations, take more medications, and use more health care facilities than men. Although many infirmities are part and parcel of aging, the woman who strives to protect her health in middle age, not to mention at a younger age, is that much more assured of living a longer, disease-free life.

If you are one of the 10 to 25 percent of women in this country who experience menopausal symptoms severe enough to warrant special attention, understanding those symptoms and the wide range of treatment options can help you overcome your difficulties. For the many others—60 to 75 percent of women—who experience milder physical symptoms, understanding the changes your body is undergoing can help you gain perspective and appreciate menopause for what it is: a perfectly natural occurrence.

> "I've always had a tendency to listen to my body and its changes, especially after having five children and two miscarriages. When I turned 50, I began having night sweats and heart palpitations. Yet I felt really terrific. I wondered what was going on, until it occurred to me that maybe menopause was responsible. I started going into bookstores and looking for information. Once I started reading about menopause, I felt so much more reassured about the things I was experiencing."

For all women—even the estimated 15 percent who will glide through menopause without notice—an awareness of the hormonal changes that accompany menopause can spark a new respect for your body. No matter which category you fall into, this book is intended to help you understand the menopausal transition and your post-menopausal options so that you can make the health decisions that are right for you.

I'd like to point out at the start of this guide that I personally don't think of menopause as a medical condition; nor should you. As stated, it is a natural passage that sometimes gives rise to symptoms that can benefit from medical, or nonmedical, treatment. And it also appears to trigger certain longer-term systemic changes, such as bone loss, which some women may need to treat. Yet menopause itself is as natural a transition as puberty.

As a doctor in a large patient-care hospital, I see a lot of women with health needs associated with menopause. I'm glad I can help them address those concerns, but let's not "medicalize" menopause. I never forget that the women I *don't* see are the majority—the women passing through menopause who don't need special care. This book, then, gives a description of what all women can expect from menopause, and also speaks to the minority who may need care. The danger in writing such a book is that readers may get the idea that menopause *requires* medical treatment, when very often it doesn't. Nonetheless, even if your menopause presents hardly any symptoms, this is an important stage in life and you should let your doctor know it's occurring. This can help him or her keep track of your overall health profile.

I've written this book to answer as fully as possible the questions and concerns that women facing menopause have brought to me. Understanding how your body works will help you make the best decisions to safeguard your health.

What Is Menopause?

Menopause is defined as the time when a woman's menses, or menstruation, permanently ceases. After menopause, a woman will no longer ovulate—that is, produce eggs that can be fertilized to develop into a baby. Although much remains to be known about why menopause occurs, it appears to be closely tied to the depletion of follicles, tiny cellular entities found in the ovaries. Each follicle is made up of an egg surrounded by cells. Surprisingly, a woman's number of eggs begins diminishing even before she is born. The ovaries of a 20-week-old female embryo hold a few million eggs. By birth, the number falls to 700,000

Figure 1. Female Reproductive System, Side View

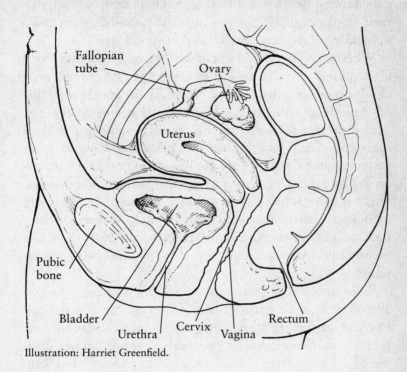

Illustration: Harriet Greenfield.

and continues to wane until only a few thousand eggs, at most, survive at menopause. Only on rare occasions has pregnancy been known to occur in the first few years after menopause.

Follicles produce estrogen, the all-important hormone which, along with the hormone progesterone, plays a key role in producing and regulating your monthly pattern of menstruation. As you age and your eggs die off, your ovaries' production of estrogen in turn diminishes. Researchers suspect that this loss of estrogen is responsible for many of menopause's associated symptoms and physical changes, notably hot flashes, vaginal atrophy (deterioration of vaginal tissue), and the body's increased vulnerability to osteoporosis and heart disease.

Whether you've had ten children or none, menopause's arrival appears to be linked to your age rather than your childbearing activity. The average age of menopause for an American woman is 51.3, plus or minus five years. Many pregnancies do not necessarily make for a later menopause. Smoking, researchers have found, consistently results in an earlier menopause by one to two years, on average. To speculate, this may result from smoking's toxic effect on the follicles and estrogen production. An early menopause also can result from a family history of early menopausal transitions. Similarly, a family history of late menopauses can account for a later-than-usual menopause.

Since age acts as the major determinant of menopause's arrival, it may be nature's way of not allowing a woman to conceive too far past her prime, in case she cannot sustain a healthy pregnancy or properly rear her young. Writing in the journal *Menopause,* Dr. John Franklin Donaldson advanced this idea by proposing that human menopause might have evolved in response to changing

"I'm 56 and haven't undergone menopause. In fact, my periods are as regular as they were thirty years ago. My doctor's told me not to be alarmed, that a late menopause can be the sign of a healthy constitution—or it can be inherited. My doctor's mentioned, however, that the later menopause is, the longer certain tissue—like breast tissue—will be exposed to higher levels of estrogen. For some women, that may translate into a slightly increased risk of breast cancer."

terrestrial conditions some 2.5 million years ago. As early humans underwent the change from a tropical rain forest habitat to biseasonal ground life, more frequent dry seasons might have led to increased mortality rates. Menopause, by cutting short a woman's reproductive life, would have allowed her to have fewer children, thus safeguarding her own health. Also, the cessation of menses would have allowed her time to better sustain the nourishment and growth of those children she bore.

In the same issue of *Menopause*, Dr. Frederick Naftolin, Patricia Whitten, and Dr. David Keefe proposed a different theory regarding menopause's evolutionary origins. As they pointed out, many menopausal symptoms and conditions mimic puerperium, the weeks following childbirth. The mother's lowered estrogen provokes genital atrophy. Lowered estrogen also leads to hot flashes that provide heat to help keep the baby warm, the rerouting/loss of calcium that goes into milk production, and poor sleep quality that keeps the mother more vigilant. Menopause, then, could be described as a final, more exaggerated puerperium period, the authors suggested.

A small minority of women—an estimated 1 to 4 percent—undergo menopause before the age of 40. Referred to as "premature" menopause, such instances can be caused by autoimmune and endocrine disorders or childhood illnesses such as mumps or viral infections. Doctors speculate that an earlier than normal menopause may also be caused by inherited factors such as an inherited propensity for ovaries that contain fewer than normal follicles. Other circumstances that can influence an early (albeit, nonnatural) menopause include malnourishment, chemotherapy, radiation treatment, and pelvic surgery.

Most women can expect to experience a "natural"

According to Dr. Kathryn Martin, an MGH endocrinologist, "Many of the cases of premature ovarian failure that we see have no obvious cause. When we're able to pinpoint a cause, the most common are chromosomal abnormalities, autoimmune problems, and chemotherapy."

menopause—that is, one that arrives on its own schedule and isn't triggered by medical intervention. A premature menopause, although pushed forward by an inherited or disease-caused event, is still considered natural. A "surgical" menopause, on the other hand, is considered nonnatural and occurs when both ovaries are removed to treat cancer, endometriosis, or some other medical problem. This results in an immediate menopause. Similarly, in some cases chemotherapy and radiation treatment can also inadvertently cause a nonnatural ovarian failure and permanent loss of menstruation.

"I got my period when I was 13. By the time I turned 16, it had stopped. The doctor I went to see was really humiliating. He kept asking if I could be pregnant and gave me a pregnancy test even after I said I'd never been sexually active. I was put on thyroid medication, but my period didn't return. I had exploratory surgery at age 18, and a new doctor said he thought one ovary had never worked and the other had just stopped working. A lot of people have searched for a quick and easy answer as to why, but an answer has never been found."

As will be further explained in Chapter 2, a hysterectomy that removes only the uterus but leaves one or both ovaries intact *does not interfere with the arrival of a natural menopause*. Although menstruation will cease because of the lack of a uterus, the operation will not induce

Figure 2. Female Reproductive System, Front View

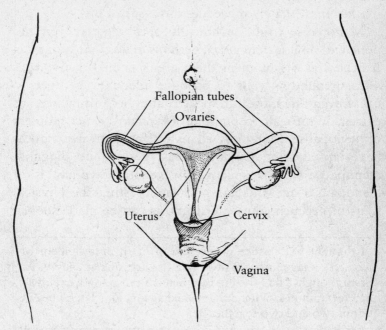

Illustration: Harriet Greenfield.

menopause, since the ovaries will continue producing hormones. In this one case only, therefore, the cessation of menses in not equated with menopause. However, for some women, removal of the uterus can contribute to an earlier than usual ovarian failure further along in time.

What Is Perimenopause?

If you're in your mid-forties and start noticing changes in your menstrual cycles or experiencing hot flashes, you're apt to believe that menopause has arrived. In fact, if the detected changes are indeed menopause-related, what has started isn't menopause, but *perimenopause*, the years or months immediately preceding this stage of life.

Menopause itself, technically speaking, is over and done with in less than a day, perhaps in less than a minute. It occurs at the moment there aren't enough active eggs and surrounding cells to produce adequate estrogen to cause even one more full menstrual cycle. In practice, it's extremely difficult to pinpoint a woman's exact moment of menopause. Many physicians wait until twelve months have lapsed after a woman's last period and diagnose menopause in retrospect. However, if a woman is of menopausal age and has been manifesting the physical signs of perimenopause, a diagnosis can be made sooner.

> "I thought hot flashes were either a myth or a figment of women's imagination—until I had my first one at age 49. At first I thought I had the flu. But then the sensation went away in a few minutes. When it happened again a day later, I began to put two and two together."

For many women, irregular bleeding will be the first telltale sign that perimenopause has begun and that menopause is nearing. Gradually you realize that your once punctual period is more erratic. Reduced amounts of estrogen and progesterone can no longer support the even monthly buildup and slough-off of cells along the uterine wall, a process so central to keeping the uterus viable for pregnancy. Hormonal irregularities translate into menstrual irregularities. Usually perimenopause starts in the mid- to late forties and typically lasts four years. Some 10 percent of menopausal women, however, abruptly cease their periods, bypassing any signs of perimenopause.

A small minority of others ride out perimenopause and its symptoms for up to six years, occasionally even longer.

> "For me, menopause and hot flashes seem to have arrived simultaneously, without any lead-up. Ever since I began getting hot flashes, I haven't had a period."

As is true of menopause in general, perimenopause's repercussions vary greatly from individual to individual. You may experience shorter or longer intervals between periods, or the periods themselves may become shorter or longer, lighter or heavier. It's not uncommon for cycles to shrink or expand beyond the normal cycle range of 21 to 35 days.

> "When I was 49, what signaled that menopause was coming was that I began getting very long periods, up to twelve days in duration. I had to cancel engagements, because the flow could be so heavy. If I laughed or sneezed, it was like a dam broke."

Be aware, however, that perimenopause coincides with a time in women's lives when the incidence of pelvic disorders are statistically high. Irregular bleeding may not be menopause-related, but an indication instead of any one of a number of medical problems. Heavy bleeding, for instance, can signal the presence of *fibroids*—noncancerous tumors—in the uterus. Most fibroids, however, cause no symptoms. (An extremely common condition, fibroids occur in close to 50 percent of women near the age of 50.) Heavy discharge can also be a sign of endometrial polyps, cancerous tissue, or precancerous conditions, among other disorders. This is why it's so tremendously important to report any menstrual irregularities to your doctor.

> "What I thought was menopause wasn't menopause at all. It turned out to be a lawyer."

If your menstrual cycles cease, it may not necessarily mean you're entering menopause; you could be pregnant! (Although pregnancy at age 50 is quite rare, pregnancy at age 40 is becoming more common.) Loss of bleeding, or *amenorrhea,* can also be caused by malnourishment, overexercise, stress, thyroid or adrenal gland abnormalities, or *prolactinoma,* a benign pituitary tumor. Usually reversible with treatment, amenorrhea need not affect menopause's natural time of arrival.

Menopause in Our Times

Within the animal kingdom, only humans routinely undergo menopause. But scientists speculate that if other primates that also menstruate (namely all Old World monkeys and apes) were to live as long as humans, certain of these species might also reach menopause. In 1981 two elderly chimpanzees, aged 48 and 50, were studied at the Yerkes Regional Primate Research Center at Emory University. They displayed hormonal changes similar to those found in perimenopausal women but died a few years later before manifesting menopause.

It used to be that, like today's Old World monkeys and apes, most female *Homo sapiens* didn't live beyond their reproductive years. (Bear in mind that this reflects only the average. Some women far outlived menopause.) As Elizabeth W. Markson, a gerontologist at Boston University, has observed: "It is only during the twentieth century that average life expectancy has markedly increased, especially in industrialized nations. When Julius Caesar was born some two thousand years ago, average life expectancy at birth was only about 22 years. . . . At the time Lincoln was elected to the presidency in the nineteenth century, life expectancy at birth had increased to perhaps 42 years. Even in 1900 life expectancy at birth was age 49." *Average* life expectancy in centuries past was all the lower because of high infant mortality rates. As for those who lived into adulthood, studies of adult skeletons of the ancient Greeks indicate an average life expectancy of 45 years—still far lower than today.

A woman born in the United States in 1993 can now expect to live an average of 78.9 years, a man 72 years, according to the National Center for Health Statistics. Moreover, the woman who reached age 65 in 1990 can expect on average to live another 18 years, to age 83. Although our potential life span may remain fixed at 110 to 120 years, as many scientists believe, our new ability to fulfill more of those years is likely due to a combination of advances, including lower infant and maternal mortality rates; new vaccines, antibiotics, and specialized drugs; control over many infectious diseases; sanitation and public health improvements; and better diet.

Consequently, while the majority of women once didn't live to see menopause, today the majority not only live through it but live nearly three decades beyond it. "Today, death before age 65 is unusual in this country," notes Markson. (The U.S. Census reports that in 1990, 36,000 Americans were over the age of 100. It could be that, as a society, we need to revise our idea of "old age"; certainly menopause can no longer be considered a precursor to senility, as it was sometimes viewed in the past.) With a greater number of women experiencing menopause and living decades beyond it, it seems small wonder that many are examining it on a personal level and using it as a marker in time for preventive care for the future.

If life expectancy has increased, does that mean that the age of menopause has gotten later? It is well documented that in this country the average age of menarche has fallen from 16 to 12.5 over the last one hundred and fifty years. The reason is better diet and therefore more rapid physical development, say researchers. As for the average age of menopause, many claim that it hasn't changed since antiquity. Other researchers, however, report that in populations where diet has noticeably improved, the average age of menopause is arriving later than it used to.

While this population trend has not been widely studied, on an individual basis overweight women have been shown to commonly undergo a late menopause, whereas very thin women are candidates for an early menopause. Researchers have observed that the undernourished Kalahari woman in Africa reaches menarche at the relatively late age of 16 and menopause at the early age of 45. The mean age of menopause for a Pakistani woman is 47, investigators report, while the average age for a Mayan woman in Chichimila, Mexico, is 44.

Menopause in Different Cultures

As a small cadre of researchers is finding, a woman's economic and cultural environment can influence the biological mechanism underlying menopause and its symptoms, as well as how a woman perceives menopause and reacts to her symptoms.

Reports of hot flashes, night sweats, and other menopausal symptoms vary from culture to culture. For instance, compared to the 75 percent of American women who reportedly experience hot flashes, a 1993 study of menopausal Mayan women from the Mexican village of Chichimila recorded no complaints of hot flashes. A 1986 study of menopausal women in Central Java conducted by anthropologist Marcha Flint cited that only 7 to 22 percent recalled hot flashes. Could it be that women who report few or no hot flashes aren't undergoing the same midlife hormonal changes that women in this country undergo? In the Mayan study, researchers from the University of California/San Francisco confirmed the same amount of estrogen loss as seen in American postmenopausal women, suggesting a comparable ovarian change.

If midlife women everywhere experience the same hormonal changes, why do reports of hot flashes vary so among populations? The answer might lie in a culture's positive or negative perception of menopause, according to Flint and other researchers. In 1965, when Flint interviewed 483 women belonging to India's Rajput caste and heard no mention of hot flashes, she speculated that the lack of complaint about these symptoms might be tied to the fact that Rajput women have more to look forward to after menopause. As younger women, their activities are restricted, since their culture views the menstruating woman as impure and inferior. After menopause, they socialize more and gain more respect. Similarly, for the Mayan women in Chichimila who reported no hot flashes, "Menopause is welcomed as a favorable transition to a new niche in the village lifestyle, characterized by relief from childbearing, acceptance as a respected elder, and a surrendering of many household chores," UCSF researchers reported.

Many nonindustrialized cultures—the Yanomamo of South America, the Bantu of South Africa, the Moroccans, the Bengali, and the Chinese, to name a few—place limitations on younger women. Menopause often brings an elevated status within the family and community, greater kindness and consideration, leadership possibilities and, in general, more freedom of expression and mobility. In numerous African, Asian, Mexican, and South American societies, older women gain considerable prestige and power. Exactly to what degree women in these societies sublimate menopausal symptoms in anticipation of better years ahead requires further study, however.

In Japan, where older women are revered more than younger women, the incidence of hot flashes is reportedly 20 percent lower than in the United States. Aside from whatever cultural attitudes may be affecting this lower rate, recent research brings to light another possible explanation. Unlike the typical high-fat Western diet, the lower-fat Japanese diet contains far more grains and vegetables, providing higher amounts of *phyto-estrogens,* weak estrogens derived from plants. In a recent, albeit very small study, researchers discovered that Japanese women excreted 100 to 1,000 times more of these estrogens than Western women. High levels of circulating phyto-estrogens, the researchers suggested, might partly explain the infrequency of hot flashes and other menopausal symptoms among Japanese women. Any direct causative relationship between plant estrogens and reduced menopausal symptoms is far from proven. It's interesting to note, however, that herbalists propose that the phyto-estrogens in certain herbs can help to quell menopausal symptoms. (See Section Three for a further discussion of alternative menopausal treatments.)

While many cultures perceive the end of a woman's reproductive life as a positive milestone, others have historically looked upon this ending with disappointment, even disdain. There is little research on how a society's negative perception of menopause might influence its population's menopausal symptoms. However, on an individual basis, women who enter menopause anticipating the worst from it are more likely to complain of symptoms than women who approach it with fewer apprehensions, according to the Massachusetts Women's Health Study and another study by researchers at the University of Pittsburgh.

> "In your forties, you keep hearing about how horrible menopause is . . . the big, black cloud ahead. But, you know, it wasn't bad at all."

Past generations in Western societies, in particular, gave vent to the view that menopause spelled both the end of the "fruitful" part of a woman's existence and the onset of mental instability. Writing on "Cultural Models for Coping with Menopause," author Joyce Griffen quoted an earlier 1969 study: " 'It is commonly believed that the menopause can induce insanity; in order to ward it off, some [rural Irish] women have retired from life in their mid-forties and, in at least three contemporary cases, have confined themselves to bed until death years later.' " A footnote by Griffen adds: "This belief also appears in rural northern New England." To be sure, such beliefs reflect the thinking of past eras. Although we in this country have largely dispelled the false rumors associated with menopause, how far have we actually come in accepting menopause's connection to aging? Jonathan Swift's observation that "Every man desires to live long, but no man would be old" seems as valid today as it was over two centuries ago.

Menopause in America

In former generations of women, the topic of menopause was largely considered unmentionable. As a rule, our mothers, grandmothers, and great-grandmothers were more highly valued as childbearers, so their status fell when their reproductive years ran out. As the dividing line, menopause was an easy target for disparagement. Wulf Utian, founding president of the North American Menopause Society, has noted that negative attitudes toward menopause had crept into Western medical and nonmedical literature by the 1700s. As late as 1935, menopause was still being referred to as the "dangerous age" that could lead to a woman's downfall. Given menopause's poor reputation, what woman would want to talk about it or admit to undergoing it?

> "A few decades ago," a 72-year-old woman recalls, "the word 'menopause' never came up outside the doctor's office, and rarely inside. It simply was something that happened to your period—or your 'curse.' Ugh, what a word!"

For those women who experienced severe menopausal symptoms, no precedent existed that encouraged them to seek medical assistance. In their day, obstetrics and women's health focused almost exclusively on pregnancy, birth, and the health of mother and baby. In the field of obstetrics and gynecology, no organized care existed for older women—another reason why earlier generations may have internalized or downplayed their menopausal transition.

In this country, a growing acceptance of menopause is decidedly helping to ease earlier negative attitudes. Yet the former stereotypical claim—that menopause is a time to be dreaded—dies hard. Younger women, in particular, tend to harbor more negative feelings toward menopause, even though studies suggest that women who have made the transition generally remember it as a time of no great hardship. In 1990, using data derived from the Massachusetts Women's Health Study, researchers at the New England Research Institutes cited that over 70 percent of women reported relief or neutral feelings about their menopausal transition, while only 2.7 percent reported regret.

> "I don't miss my period one bit. Who likes sitting around on a wet pad!"

Nonetheless, the stigma of menopause will probably never entirely disappear until, as a society, we grow old more gracefully and face death more acceptingly. As the large baby-boom generation moves toward age 50, we appear to be making room for a new focus on capable, healthy older women. Magazines and television are paying more attention to middle-aged and older people and catering to their energy and interests. Yet "there are some real confusions going on," observes Marcha Flint. "We're living longer and pushing back old age well beyond menopause. But we're still essentially a youth-oriented society that glamorizes youth and shuts out aging."

As hard as it may be to accept growing older, unlike previous generations, you have more time to acclimate to your later years and to ensure that they are as healthy as possible. Menopause can become an important adjustment point. While there's no escaping the fact that you can't live forever, today you at least have numerous options that can help prevent the stroke at age 65 or the bone fracture at 70. This book will help you not only manage any troublesome symptoms of menopause, but also attain your goals for a healthier later life.

Part One

Menopause and
Its Effects

1

What Causes Menopause?

During midlife, a woman—unlike a man—experiences very noticeable hormonal changes. Aging is the major instigator of these changes. As a woman grows older, her ovaries reduce their store of eggs, which in turn influences signals received and emitted by the brain that have a bearing on the endocrine system's yield of female hormones. This chain of events, which ultimately results in menopause, picks up speed in your mid- to late thirties, although you may not begin noticing related symptoms for another decade or so.

The Endocrine System

Made up of nearly a dozen organs, the endocrine system produces many different types of chemical messengers—hormones—that are vital to the body's development and maintenance. In both sexes, certain endocrine organs, or glands, are instrumental in developing and sustaining sex-related characteristics and functions. These glands include: the hypothalamus at the base of the brain; the kidney-bean-sized pituitary gland tucked right below the hypothalamus; the ovaries in the female and the testes in the male; and, to a lesser extent, the adrenal glands, which are perched atop the kidneys.

We tend to think of our bodies in terms of flesh, blood, and bone. Yet no bodily function as we know it could occur without the constant chemical messages delivered by hormones. Released by a gland in one part of the body, these organic molecules get swept through the blood to organs and tissues in other parts of the body, where each conveys a specific message. For instance, were it not for hormones released by the ovaries, the endometrial lining wouldn't be built up and shed each month, nor could an embryo form and develop.

Estrogen

Certain hormones produced by both women and men are referred to as "female hormones" because they are devoted primarily to biological tasks largely unique to the female. Of these, estrogen is the most prominent in the human female. Men produce far lower quantities of female hormones than women do, just as women—whose bodies also make male hormones, including testosterone—produce far less of these male-oriented substances in comparison to men.

Dubbed the "feminizing hormone," estrogen plays a pivotal role in the early maturation of the vagina, uterus, Fallopian tubes, and other female organs, as well as secondary sex characteristics such as the enlargement of breasts and hips. In concert with progesterone, another female hormone made by the ovaries, estrogen issues the instructions that sustain each menstrual cycle and prepare the uterus for pregnancy.

Over 90 percent of the estrogen that circulates in a premenopausal woman's body is made in the ovaries. The adrenal glands account for much smaller amounts. So do peripheral tissues such as fat, liver, and kidneys, which convert a female's male hormones, collectively known as androgens, to estrogens. Because the hormone is produced in small amounts by these other sources, postmenopausal women are not totally lacking in estrogen. Also, because of the estrogen converted by androgens in fat cells, overweight women may suffer less from menopause-related problems, such as hot flashes and osteoporosis, which are related to estrogen depletion. Yet they can be more at risk for diseases that have been linked to estrogen output, such as endometrial and breast cancer. Researchers have shown that because overweight woman have less of the protein SHBG, "sex hormone-binding globulin," which serves as a carrier for estrogen, less estrogen is bound to SHBG. Therefore more estrogen remains more active or potent within their systems.

Women, it's been discovered, actually have dozens of types of circulating estrogens. Only three of these—*estradiol, estrone,* and *estriol*—circulate in significant quantities and potencies. Before menopause, when estrogen levels are their highest, the predominant circulating estrogen is estradiol, the most potent natural estrogen. After menopause, when estrogen is reduced, estrone is most in evidence. Estriol, made from a combination of components from the placenta, fetus, and mother, comes into play mostly during pregnancy.

Even though levels of estrone may actually rise after menopause, postmenopausal estrone is insufficient in quantity and activity to override the functional loss of estradiol, according to MGH research endocrinologist David T. MacLaughlin. The loss of total estrogen activity is evidenced by resulting symptoms and changes, such as hot flashes and bone loss.

Overall, many different sources of estrogens can affect the human body. First, there are those made by the body, as well as mostly synthetic estrogens produced by pharmaceutical companies. Shaped in the laboratory, yet closely similar in their molecular structure to naturally occurring estrogens, these prepared estrogens are referred to as *exogenous* (that is, they are introduced into the body from without). Exogenous estrogens, as well as exogenous progestins and androgens, are used for *hormone replacement therapy* (HRT)—the medical practice of putting ovarian hormones back into the body to replace those lost to menopause.

There are also a broad category of *xenoestrogens,* estrogenlike compounds linked to sources other than humans and animals. Similar to human estrogens, xenoestrogens can reportedly attach to human estrogen receptors and thereby influence estrogen-receptive tissues and organs. Some xenoestrogens—phyto-estrogens from plants, for example—may directly affect existing estrogen levels.

Researchers once thought that the estrogen made by the body affected only the uterus. In fact, this versatile hormone accounts for much more than a woman's strictly female traits. After estrogen leaves the ovaries, it travels to estrogen-specific receptors, or receiving points, found in different type tissues all over the body. As might be expected, many of these receptors are present in female attributes, such as the breast, uterus, labia, and vulva. Yet they also reside in bone, skin, the brain, muscles, heart, and blood vessels. Estrogen usually influences the tissues it penetrates in positive ways: by lessening factors tied to cardiovascular disease and bone loss, for instance. When menopause's decline of estrogenic activity occurs, estrogen-sensitive cells lose some of their resiliency. Estrogen depletion can be the culprit behind increasingly brittle bone that's susceptible to fracture. It also may partially explain why a woman's risk for heart disease increases after menopause.

Soon after 1942, when laboratory-prepared estrogen first became available in pill form, it was hailed all too hastily as a youth-prolonging elixir. Although estrogen can have a protective effect on health, estrogen taken in excess or metabolized by the body in a certain way can create problems. As far back as the 1930s and 1940s, research demonstrated that large or prolonged doses of estrogen can cause breast tumors in rats and carcinoma in the cervix of mice.

Even mild estrogenlike compounds present in plants can trigger adverse reactions when an animal gets too much of them. For example, pigs that eat too much moldy corn and sheep that overindulge on clover can display an abnormal growth of the uterine lining, high miscarriage rates, and other abnormalities associated with an excessive exposure to estrogen-mimicking hormones.

Other xenoestrogens may indirectly increase or decrease "good" and "bad" estrogens in our body. Some scientists speculate, for instance, that estrogenlike chlorinated compounds found in pesticides, by binding to human estrogen receptors, may increase both men's and women's risk for cancer.

A recent theory by researchers at the Strang-Cornell Cancer Research Laboratory in New York proposes that the way estrogen is metabolized in the body may influence the incidence rate of hormonally related cancers, such as breast and endometrial cancer. "All ovarian-made estrogen is metabolized by one of two principle pathways," according to Strang-Cornell investigator H. Leon Bradlow. One pathway results in a "good" estrogen (2-hydroxyestrone); the other leads to a bad, cancer-causing estrogen (16-alpha hydroxyestrone). Many different factors can affect the metabolic pathway, from inherited features, diet, and thyroid hormones, to the presence of xenoestrogens such as pesticide residues, according to Bradlow.

What the whole picture suggests is that estrogens originating from several sources can pose benefits or risks. There is the body's natural output of estrogens, which can be normal or abnormal; there are the possible influences of estrogen replacement supplements to consider; and there is the possible further influence of estrogens found in the environment around us. While the pros and cons of hormone replacement will be reviewed in Chapter 6, it should be noted that estrogen supplements alone don't necessarily pose the only risks and benefits for users. A woman's inherited makeup, current health, diet, and surrounding environment may all play a part in her body's reaction to estrogen.

Progestin

Progesterone is the second most significant female hormone. Two types of progestin—pure progesterone and a derivative—are made primarily by the ovaries, with smaller amounts secreted by the adrenals. Devoted primarily to tasks necessary for reproduction, this hormone stimulates the growth of a cushiony endometrial lining that serves as a nest for the fertilized egg, prepares breast tissue for the secretion of breast milk, and generally maintains the advancement of pregnancy. Although progesterone receptors are found mostly in reproductive organs, researchers have also found them in bone and in certain areas of the brain, where their function is still unclear.

Androgen

Small amounts of male hormones, known collectively as *androgens,* circulate in the female before and after menopause. While the role that male hormones play in women is subtle and requires further study, these chemical messengers are absorbed by many different types of cells all over the body, the same way estrogens are. They are thought to enhance sexual desire, contribute to sexual functioning, and may heighten energy levels and a sense of well-being. Absorbed by bone cells, they contribute to bone growth. They possibly also contribute to brain functioning, eye lubrication, and many other as yet dimly realized functions. Those androgens most in evidence are testosterone, androstenedione, and dehydroepiandrosterone.

Although androgens are produced in equal amounts by the ovaries and adrenal glands, they are also converted from biologically inactive "prehormone" steroids found in the skin, liver, brain, muscle, and other tissues. The body converts some androgen into the estrogen estrone, which helps to make up for the loss of ovarian-made estrogen after menopause.

In comparison to the 70 to 80 percent decrease in total circulating estrogen that occurs with menopause, androgen levels decline by only 10 to 50 percent. Still, because of the higher relative ratio of androgen to estrogen after menopause, some women acquire more facial hair, a deeper voice, and other androgen-accentuated characteristics.

A Normal Menstrual Cycle

Your menstrual cycle depends upon the intricate and delicate interplay between the hypothalamus, pituitary, ovaries

Figure 3. Menstrual Cycle

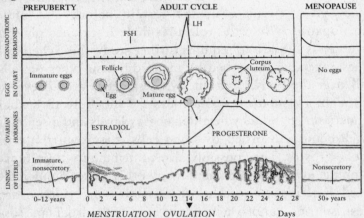

Shortly before a girl reaches puberty, her pituitary gland begins to secrete more follicle-stimulating hormone (FSH) and luteinizing hormone (LH). Menstruation begins when LH is produced in a steady, rhythmic pattern and in sufficient quantities. Periods normally recur in a cyclic pattern as these hormones work in concert with estradiol and progesterone.

During the first half of the menstrual cycle, LH and FSH are secreted at steady levels and stimulate the ovary to produce a mature egg. At midcycle, there is a sudden surge of both LH and FSH, causing the ovary to release the egg (ovulation). Just as abruptly, FSH and LH levels drop to their baseline levels.

Immediately prior to ovulation, the ovary steps up its production of estradiol. After egg release, there is an increase in progesterone, which is produced by the corpus luteum. These hormones act together to promote endometrial growth. If an egg is not fertilized and/or does not implant in the uterus, estradiol and progesterone levels fall, the endometrium is sloughed, and menstruation ensues. Just prior to the end of the cycle, FSH levels slowly start to rise, beginning the cycle again.

Illustration: Harriet Greenfield; caption: Harvard Medical School Health Publications Group.

Figure 4. Menstrual Cycle and Hormone Interactions

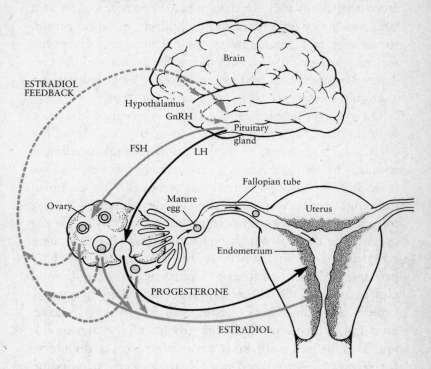

Hormones produced in different parts of the body interact to produce a woman's menstrual cycles. The pituitary gland secretes follicle-stimulating hormone (FSH) and luteinizing hormone (LH). In response to FSH, an egg maturing in the ovary produces estradiol, the rise of which stimulates increased output of LH and FSH. At its peak level, LH causes the follicle enclosing the egg to rupture; it releases the egg and begins to produce progesterone. Working together, progesterone and estradiol ready the endometrium for implantation while suppressing release of FSH and LH.

Illustration: Harriet Greenfield;
caption: Harvard Medical School Health Publications Group.

and uterus. The recurring monthly pattern of hormone and tissue changes prepares both an egg for fertilization and the uterus for pregnancy. In days when menarche began at a later age and women had more children, it was common for women to have as few as one hundred fifty cycles before menopause. Today, with menarche earlier and the tendency of women to have fewer children, it's not unusual for a woman to undergo as many as four hundred.

On average the menstrual cycle lasts twenty-eight days, with the first day of bleeding traditionally considered the cycle's starting point, or day 1. As menstrual bleeding is ending, the hypothalamus stimulates the pituitary to release *FSH*—*f*ollicle-*s*timulating *h*ormone. This chemical messenger sets into motion the cascade of events leading to ovulation, which occurs, on average, on day 14 of the cycle. (The time of ovulation varies greatly among menstruating women.) When it reaches the ovary, FSH prompts as many as fifteen to twenty egg-containing follicles to mature. Of these, one follicle will mature more rapidly than the others. As the follicle grows, it releases estradiol, which stimulates the growth of the uterine lining. This growth is the body's way of preparing the uterus for receipt of a fertilized egg. Near the cycle's midpoint, high levels of estradiol feed back to the hypothalamus, which instructs the pituitary to release *LH*—*l*uteinizing *h*ormone. This LH surge acts on the ovary, causing continued cell division and prompting the follicle to ovulate, or release the matured egg, which is then picked up by the Fallopian tube.

The now-empty follicle, still under the influence of LH, continues growing and forms the corpus luteum. As this "yellow body" gets larger, it synthesizes significant amounts of progesterone, which further prepares the endometrium, or uterine lining, so that a fertilized egg will have a good place to land, grow, and be nourished. Meanwhile, the combination of progesterone and estrogen inhibits the secretion of further FSH and LH. If the ovulated egg is not fertilized by a male's sperm, the corpus luteum will degenerate. The hormone associated with pregnancy—*h*CG, or *h*uman *c*horionic gonadotropin—will not be produced and pregnancy will not result. The ovaries' hormone production ceases for the duration of the cycle, and the menstrual flow discards the unneeded endometrial lining. By day 28, the absence of ovarian hormones registers on the brain, which triggers a fresh surge of FSH and a new cycle.

If, instead, the ovulated egg is fertilized and you become pregnant, then production of hCG ensures that the corpus luteum remains intact and continues generating the hormones that will sustain the endometrium and the pregnancy until the placenta forms and takes over this task.

If you're born with as many follicles and eggs as you'll ever have, why doesn't your menstrual cycle begin at the time of birth? A girl doesn't reach menarche or have the ability to become pregnant until her hypothalamus has fully matured and has the ability to signal the pituitary to release its hormones. This happens just before puberty.

It's interesting to note how, in the late 1950s, scientists at the Worcester Foundation for Experimental Biology in Shrewsbury, Massachusetts, used their knowledge of the menstrual cycle to develop the world's first birth control pill. They realized that if you turn off FSH and LH, eggs can't mature and ovulate. The Pill's content of estrogen and progesterone convinces the brain that it doesn't have to initiate any new waves of FSH or LH, since estrogen and progesterone register in the system. In comparison,

"I'll get a bad headache, sleep fitfully for a night or two, not feel like communicating and end up wondering what's going on. Once I realize that it's because PMS has struck again, I feel better for the knowing."

RU 486—the French drug that is used both as a contraceptive and an abortive agent—works by blocking the pregnancy-maintaining action of progesterone on the uterus and the brain.

In a twenty-eight-day cycle, your estrogen levels rise and peak during the first two weeks, while progesterone levels remain low. During the last two weeks, while estrogen levels remain fairly high, progesterone rises and peaks. As many women are aware, fluctuating hormones—even during a normal menstrual cycle—appear to account for mood swings. Estrogen has been observed to be a mood enhancer, progesterone a mood diminisher. Correspondingly, women have reported feeling their best just before ovulation (day 14), when estrogen levels crest. Yet, as progesterone returns to the brain toward the cycle's end, it can cause tension or depression and irritability commonly known as PMS, or premenstrual syndrome, in some women. Estrogen and progesterone affect mood, endocrinologists suspect, through their modification of neurotransmitters in the brain.

What Happens As Your Ovaries Age?

Exactly why the millions of your ovarian eggs should decrease in number and activity over the years and stop functioning altogether by the end of your fifth decade remains one of the mysteries of the poorly understood aging process. Better understood are the hormonal changes that underlie menopause, particularly those involving FSH and estrogen.

When you're younger and FSH signals the follicles to make estrogen in preparation for ovulation, there are plenty of active follicles to respond. As you age, however, there are fewer and fewer follicles available for ovulation. In reaction, your pituitary secretes higher and higher levels of FSH in an attempt to stimulate what follicles remain. Think of the brain as a thermostat, the ovaries as a furnace, and the eggs as fuel. It's cold in your living room because, unknown to you, your furnace (the ovaries) has run out of fuel (the eggs). Your pituitary/brain thermostat keeps sending out more and more messages (FSH) to the furnace (the ovaries), but there's no response.

A doctor recounts, "A patient of mine was sure that the shock of her husband's death had brought on her menopause. We know that shock, or great stress, can in fact cause a shock to the hypothalamus, which can temporarily stop hormonal stimulus to the ovaries. Hence menstrual bleeding stops—a condition known as 'hypothalamic amenorrhea.' But this condition eventually always reverses, with menstrual cycles resuming."

For a long while after menopause, FSH levels remain high, until they drift lower with advanced age. Hormone supplements lower FSH only slightly. Before menopause, an ovarian hormone called *inhibin* keeps FSH in check; after menopause, inhibin's levels appear to fall, another reason for the rise in FSH. A high FSH has not been linked to any appreciable physical symptoms or physiological changes the way low amounts of estrogen have been.

How Do You Know If You're Experiencing Menopause?

If you're having irregular periods, a simple blood test that measures your FSH is the best indicator of whether or not you're menopausal. Before menopause, although FSH fluctuates, it rarely remains above 40 mIU/ml (milli international units per milliliter). A reading greater than 40 mIU/ml in the absence of several periods can indicate you're undergoing menopause. However, because FSH levels can seesaw greatly before menopause, one high reading isn't necessarily a certain sign of menopause. If you've skipped two periods, you might still ovulate in the third month. However, if you've skipped six periods, are undergoing menopausal symptoms, *and* have a high FSH reading, you are probably experiencing menopause.

Although your estrogen and LH levels can also be measured through blood tests, these measurements do not always provide a reliable picture of your menopausal status. Because premenopausal estrogen levels can be low at certain times during your menstrual cycle, a low estrogen reading doesn't necessarily signal menopause.

Often, the symptoms heralding menopause may be so obvious to a woman and her doctor that taking the FSH test may be a waste of time and money. The test can be useful, however, if you're uncertain whether you've

> "I'm age 52 and I thought menopause had come because I didn't have a period for six months. Then it came back—for another six months. Now it's gone again."

"When I had my FSH tested, I did it in order to try and make a decision. My menstrual cycles were less regular. I knew I was perimenopausal and wondered if I had enough eggs left to get pregnant. The test—a simple blood-drawing—showed I wasn't yet menopausal, indicating I probably had enough eggs left. But then the relationship I was in ended, cutting short any thoughts of pregnancy. A year later I began another relationship and had my FSH tested again, again in hopes of being able to get pregnant. At that point the test showed I was menopausal."

stopped menstruating because of menopause, pregnancy, overexertion, malnourishment, or some other condition. Menopause is the only condition that stops menstrual bleeding *and* is associated with a high FSH. All other conditions that halt bleeding register a low or normal FSH.

While menopause accounts for up to a 70 to 80 percent decrease in your *total* premenopausal estrogen, the drop in estradiol—your body's most potent estrogen—is more appreciable. Before menopause, estradiol commonly fluctuates between 50 pg/ml (picograms per milliliter) at the time of your period and 300 pg/ml at ovulation. In comparison, postmenopausal levels are usually less than 20 pg/ml. In other words, after menopause, your system may contain less than 10 percent of the estradiol that formerly circulated close to ovulation time. (Compared to all that hormones do for us, their actual amount in the body is amazingly infinitesimal. Note that one picogram is equal to one-thousandth of a billionth of a gram.) As much as 35 pg/ml of estrone, the major estrogen converted from androgens, circulates after menopause. Less active than estradiol, however, estrone has less of an effect on your tissues.

It should be noted that menopausal declines in estrogen

can elicit very different responses in women in terms of physical symptoms and conditions such as hot flashes or an increased risk of heart disease. Some women's systems accommodate the estrogen loss much better than others.

In comparison to premenopausal estrogen, the progesterone and androgen present in your system before menopause circulate in much higher, though weaker amounts. A normal menstrual cycle's progesterone level after ovulation vacillates between 6,000 and 19,000 pg/ml. After menopause, progesterone levels become practically undetectable. Prior to menopause, androgen levels can rise to 1,000 pg/ml. Upon menopause, this hormone undergoes a 10 to 50 percent decline. As male-female biological differences can attest, the circulating levels of androgens differ substantially between the sexes. Take testosterone, for instance, the primary androgen in both sexes. In a premenopausal woman, an average of 250 to 900 pg/ml of testosterone circulates through the bloodstream. This amount is approximately 10 to 20 percent less than the amount of circulating testosterone found in a male of similar age.

In summary, here's a checklist of indicators that can tell you you're entering perimenopause:

• In the last several months your periods have become irregular, or you have skipped some. Your menstrual bleeding has become heavier or lighter than previously; intervals between your cycles have become shorter or longer; or your period may have become shorter or longer.
• You find yourself occasionally waking up all hot and sweaty. Some women report that they experience night

sweats before they start experiencing hot flashes during the day.

• You've begun having hot-flash sensations—a heating up of the shoulders, neck and face—or night sweats. (See Chapter 3 for more information about symptoms.)

Two combined indicators can tell you that menopause has happened:

• You haven't had a period for six months.
• A blood test has shown that your FSH levels are over 40 mIU/ml (milli international units per milliliter).

> "I had my periods every twenty-eight days, from age 15 to age 52. Then suddenly—boom!—no more periods. They vanished that quickly."

> "Menopause was the easiest thing I've ever been through. When I was 54 my period stopped for three months. Then it came back for a year. Then it stopped completely. I had no hot flashes, no other symptoms, no nothing."

2

Menopause and Hysterectomy

It's common belief that *hysterectomy,* the surgical removal of a woman's uterus, induces menopause. Not so. The loss of the uterus doesn't interfere with the ovaries or their monthly cycling of hormones—the chemical basis for a woman's reproductive life. If you've had a hysterectomy, your menstrual bleeding stops because there's no uterine lining for the hormones to act upon. But your ovaries' production of hormones will continue at premenopausal levels until ovarian function naturally wanes.

On the other hand, the removal of both your ovaries (with or without the removal of the uterus) *will* trigger an immediate menopause. Without the ovaries, your body cannot produce enough of the hormones necessary for menstruation and pregnancy. As will be discussed later in this chapter, large doses of radiation treatment to the pelvis and certain chemotherapy drugs that damage ovarian follicles can also induce menopause. In general, any circumstance—a medical intervention, an infection or disease, or bodily injury—that stops the ovaries' secretion of hormones can elicit a sudden, earlier-than-natural ovarian failure. If menopause is hastened this way, remember that

A woman from the Midwest recounts: "No one talked to me at any length about how chemotherapy for the pelvic cancer I had would probably induce menopause—which it did. A slip of paper that listed chemotherapy's possible side effects was how I found out. Immediately after my first chemo session, I began getting terrible hot flashes—so then I really knew."

it means that your body is losing a major estrogen source ahead of its natural schedule. You and your doctor will want to evaluate your vulnerability to conditions linked to estrogen depletion, especially heart disease and osteoporosis.

Hysterectomy: Then and Now

The term "hysterectomy" actually encompasses many different kinds of surgery involving the removal of the uterus and/or ovaries. Until the middle of this century, a higher percentage of women underwent hysterectomy than do women today. Before the arrival of a new generation of antibiotics, pelvic abscesses and infections were more often viewed as life-threatening and prompted such surgery. Fear of cancer and undiagnosed pelvic pain also instigated the procedure. Moreover, before tubal ligation came into practice, hysterectomy was a popular form of sterilization for women who wanted to end their childbearing years.

Today, tubal ligations have replaced hysterectomies as the primary method of sterilization in women, with 380,000 outpatient procedures performed in the United

States in 1992. A fairly safe and easy surgery, tubal ligation involves burning, cutting, or cinching both Fallopian tubes at midsection so that an egg traveling down either tube cannot interact with sperm and become fertilized. Tubal ligation, as best we know, doesn't affect menstruation or hasten the arrival of a natural menopause.

Where once the uterus was seen as a fairly expendable organ, today there is a concerted effort to preserve it and the ovaries whenever possible. After all, taking out a major organ is serious business and carries all the risks of major surgery. While reported mortality rates for non-cancer-related hysterectomies range from 6 to 38 per 10,000, the rates of perioperative complications in the 1980s ranged from 24 percent for vaginal hysterectomy to 43 percent for abdominal hysterectomy. However, most such complications are not serious.

Hysterectomies remain one of the most frequently performed types of major surgery in this country. In 1992 580,000 hysterectomies were performed. While this was down from 650,000 a decade ago, the general consensus among health professionals is that many hysterectomies are unnecessary. If you are contemplating a hysterectomy, consult with your physician to make sure an alternative approach isn't possible. A 1993 analysis of 642 hysterectomy patients by RAND, an independent nonprofit research group in Santa Monica, California, concluded that only 58 percent of elective hysterectomies were strictly necessary. The survey didn't include hysterectomies that treated cancer or uncontrolled hemorrhage. This suggests that too many patients may be unaware of the options open to them.

Should your doctor recommend a hysterectomy for a chronic condition, such as fibroid tumors, seek a second opinion. Sometimes a simpler solution might suffice, and

A woman who had an abdominal hysterectomy recounts, "The procedure really didn't feel like a difficult one. Two things can really help: Make sure you aren't pushed out of the hospital too soon, and that when you get home, you don't have too much to do. Getting enough rest in the first week was really important. In ten days I was back in the office."

"I found a hysterectomy to be very traumatic surgery. A friend told me that after she had one, she had to take a nap every afternoon for a whole year. I was shocked and thought I'd be different; I've always had a lot of energy. Well, I was mistaken. Two weeks after my hysterectomy I was back in work, but soon after I had to take a temporary leave for two months—because I was so exhausted."

it just takes a doctor with a different orientation to realize it. When strictly medically indicated, however, the operation can bring much improvement and relief of your symptoms. A recent study led by Dr. Karen J. Carlson, director of MGH's Women's Health Associates, evaluated women who had had hysterectomies to treat benign conditions. The study's results showed that a hysterectomy was "very effective for relieving symptoms and improving the quality of life for women who were quite symptomatic before surgery," said Carlson.

"The large fibroid I had threatened to cause organ damage and was causing major problems when I urinated. I can't tell you what relief my hysterectomy brought. I'm totally back to normal."

Reasons for Hysterectomy

A wide range of pelvic disorders can call for a hysterectomy. As reported by *The New England Journal of Medicine* in a 1993 review of hysterectomies written by this author and two other MGH physicians, uterine fibroid tumors account for approximately 30 percent of hysterectomies; abnormal uterine bleeding due to hormonal imbalances for 20 percent; endometriosis for another 20 percent; genital prolapse for about 15 percent; and chronic pelvic pain associated with myriad causes for approximately 10 percent. Malignant and premalignant conditions, complications of pregnancy, and advanced pelvic inflammatory disease (also known as PID) can also be legitimate reasons for a hysterectomy. In all cases, the severity of the problem dictates whether or not a hysterectomy is absolutely necessary, or if a less intrusive alternative might work.

Uterine Fibroids

Ranging from smaller than a pea to larger than a grapefruit, uterine fibroids are tumors arising from the uterus' layer of smooth muscle. Growing inside the uterine cavity, within the wall, or on the outer surface of the uterus, these tumors are usually benign, or noncancerous. Only an estimated 1 in 10,000 have been found to be malignant. Moreover, the vast majority of fibroids, known medically as *leiomyomas,* produce no symptoms. You might realize you have them only when a doctor's physical exam or an ultrasound exam administered for some other reason reveals them.

The larger the fibroid, the greater the chance you'll have symptoms. These may include heavy menstrual bleeding, pelvic pain, and lower abdominal pressure. If fibroids press on your rectum, bladder, or urethra, they can also produce severe constipation or urinary problems.

Fibroids are hardly rare in older women; close to 50 percent of women around the age of 50 have them. It's not understood why they form, nor is it clear why they cause excessive menstrual bleeding. It could be that they increase the area of the uterine lining, that the tissue overlining the fibroid might be abnormal, or that the fibroid might prevent muscles in the uterine wall from contracting and squeezing blood vessels that otherwise stop the bleeding.

When fibroids present symptoms, you may want to try to wait them out if you're close to menopausal age. Because most fibroids require estrogen for growth, most shrink naturally after menopause. A hysterectomy is usually considered only when fibroids are potentially malignant or when they are very large and cause anemia, pain, or bladder or bowel problems. If fibroids are causing infertility, recurrent miscarriage, or premature delivery in a woman intent on childbearing, a doctor will usually try to avoid a hysterectomy. The aim instead might be to detach and remove only the tumor through the vagina or abdomen. This procedure is known as a *myomectomy*.

Another option is drug therapy designed to shrink fi-

"Just recently I had a baseball-sized fibroid removed by way of a myomectomy. Using really thin tools inserted through small incisions in my abdomen, the surgeon cut the fibroid loose and cut it into pieces, which were removed through a one-inch incision at the base of my abdomen. I feel really lucky. Only a few years ago I might have been in for a hysterectomy. The fibroid had been causing changes in urination and bowel movements, and discomfort."

> A 47-year-old woman who had her uterus removed on account of a four-inch-wide attached fibroid explains the decision making she went through: "I could have simply had the fibroid itself extracted. But in my case—given the size of the fibroid and its location—it would have been a more complicated operation than having a hysterectomy. Also, my doctor told me there was a 30 percent chance of developing another fibroid. Since my childbearing years are over, removal of the uterus seemed the way to go."

broids; this can be done alone or in combination with a myomectomy. Known as *GnRH* (gonadotropin-releasing hormone) *agonists,* drugs such as leuprolide, nafarelin, and goserelin temporarily shrink fibroids by turning off the pituitary gland. This stops the ovaries from being stimulated into producing the estrogen on which fibroids thrive.

GnRH agonists carry one major disadvantage: They can shortchange a woman's system of its natural estrogen, leaving her prone to hot flashes and other symptoms of estrogen depletion and at greater risk for heart disease, osteoporosis, and other conditions linked to estrogen shortage. This is why GnRH agonists are mostly prescribed for short terms. Exploring "add-back" therapy, researchers are currently trying to combine small amounts of estrogens with GnRH agonists. If this research is successful, the right added dose of estrogens might guard women from the symptoms and risks of estrogen decline without stimulating a fibroid's growth.

It should be noted that there have been isolated reports that GnRH agonists can have negative effects on other systems such as the nervous system. However, these observations are far from proven.

A myomectomy and drug use aren't always perfect solutions for fibroids. Within months after drug treatment ceases, fibroids frequently grow back. After a myomectomy, fibroids may also develop from fibroid "seedlings" that the procedure failed to remove. Nevertheless, a myomectomy or GnRH agonists can be used as a stopgap method to ease symptoms until a woman reaches menopause. At this point, because of less circulating estrogen, fibroids may diminish in size. The amount by which fibroids actually regress after menopause is variable.

Abnormal Uterine Bleeding

Hysterectomy is sometimes recommended to treat heavy bleeding caused by abnormal hormonal activity associated with the uterus. On occasion, hysterectomy is also an option for excessive bleeding associated with fibroids, polyps, or new growths. But again, in these instances, hysterectomy should be a last resort.

Two different hormonal problems can promote abnormal uterine bleeding: The uterus's interior wall may be failing to staunch bleeding when a menstrual period is winding down, or a lack of adequate progesterone might result in excessive estrogen, causing too much growth of the uterine wall and hindering its monthly slough-off. Heavy bleeding in both cases can occur during or between menstrual periods.

Once they are sure that abnormal bleeding is not related to medical conditions such as leukemia, gynecologists employ several procedures to pin down the cause for abnormal bleeding. These include a *biopsy* (tissue sampling) of endometrial tissue, a *D&C* (dilatation and curettage) of the uterus, or a visual probe of the uterus with a hysteroscope inserted through the vagina. Ultrasound also can be used to detect fibroids and other abnormalities in the endometrium.

For bleeding caused by hormonal disorders, the first treatment of choice is drug therapy to regulate the levels of progesterone and estrogen in the body, using drugs such as oral contraceptives, *progestins* (synthetic progesterone), and GnRH agonists. Nonsteroidal anti-inflammatory drugs (such as ibuprofen or Anaprox) also can be used. Instead of influencing hormonal activity, nonsteroidal anti-inflammatory drugs act on the uterine lining. By controlling the constriction and dilation of blood vessels and muscles, they can reduce bleeding.

If drug therapy proves ineffective, *endometrial ablation* is another approach to halt bleeding. In essence, a heat source such as a laser beam or an electrically heated roller-ball is used to burn and destroy the uterine lining. Although endometrial ablation halts bleeding in a reported 70 to 90 percent of cases, it causes sterility. It can also make it difficult to detect early signs of cancer that otherwise present themselves through abnormal bleeding, since ablation may prevent endometrial-lining bleeding from being detected.

When fibroids in the uterine lining account for heavy bleeding, a vaginal procedure that makes use of a hysteroscope's telescopic lens and a wire loop can be used to cut away the fibroid.

Unfortunately, as many as 25 percent of women who experience abnormal bleeding either fail to respond to or cannot tolerate nonsurgical therapies that avoid a hysterectomy. In such cases, a hysterectomy may become necessary.

Endometriosis

This condition arises when endometrial cells from the uterine lining appear outside the uterus and cover other organs. Just as the menstrual cycle swells the cells of the uterine lining, these aberrant endometrial-like cells similarly build up. But while the uterus can flush out its excess tissue with a menstrual period, the aberrant cells' accumulated blood and tissue get trapped inside the lower pelvis.

Endometriosis can also turn up (albeit rarely) in such far-flung places as the lung and the eye, where it can damage the organ. It might be that cells of various organs can potentially transform into endometrial-like tissue, one theory proposes. It seems less likely that endometriosis occurs because cells from the uterus have migrated.

Commonly, the resulting primary symptom is pelvic pain. Discomfort is most noticeable with menstrual bleeding and intercourse. Although researchers aren't yet sure what causes the pain, it could be connected to the scar tissue produced by endometriosis, or inflammation of the *peritoneum,* the tissue that surrounds the abdomen. Occasionally endometriosis can cause irregular bleeding, usually when the condition affects the ovaries. Women who haven't had pregnancies are more apt to experience endometriosis than those who have.

Here again, hysterectomy is reserved for the most severe cases, since a number of other treatments can effectively subdue or eliminate endometriosis. As in the case of fibroids, endometriosis appears to be estrogen-dependent; after menopause its lesions may shrink or stop growing. So if the condition isn't overly severe, a woman may decide to hold off treatment in hopes that menopause will bring improvement.

If you have pelvic pain and endometriosis is suspected, nonsteroidal anti-inflammatory drugs can be used in the short term to relieve the pain. If endometriosis has been confirmed by a procedure such as laparoscopy and requires premenopausal treatment, the first choice might be progestin-dominant oral contraceptives. These carry fewer side effects and are less costly than other treatments. It may turn out, however, that oral contraceptives don't effectively control endometriosis, in which case your doctor might prescribe estrogen-suppressing drugs such as GnRH agonists. Another option is danazol, a male-like hormone. Danazol, however, can contribute to facial hair and other masculinizing side effects. And, like GnRH agonists, danazol can be costly.

As seen with their use for fibroid treatment, estrogen-suppressing drugs for endometriosis are usually prescribed for the short term because of their estrogen-robbing effects. However, a recent MGH-headed study holds out hope for a way of prescribing GnRH agonists for longer periods without contributing to osteoporosis. When treating endometriosis with GnRH agonists, the researchers found the combined used of *parathyroid hormone,* a bone-growth stimulator, worked to prevent bone loss.

If medication fails, laparoscopic surgery through the abdomen may be performed to:

1. determine if endometriosis is indeed causing the problem;
2. determine how extensive the endometriosis is;
3. treat the condition.

Once a diagnosis is made via laparoscopy, treatment—cauterizing or burning endometriosis masses as a way of stopping their growth—usually occurs at the same time.

MGH fellow Dr. Louise Lapensee reports: "Hysterectomy is the best treatment for endometriosis, but the last procedure we like to do. We resorted to it recently for a patient who had had several laparoscopies to treat severe endometriosis. Each time the condition and pain came back. So an abdominal removal of the ovaries and uterus was decided upon. If the patient goes on hormone replacement, the endometriosis isn't likely to return, although that's not 100 percent certain."

Genital Prolapse

Genital prolapse refers to the descent or sagging of tissues and organs in the pelvic region. Without its ligament support, the uterus drops lower, as can the rectum, bladder, and vagina. Exacerbated by aging and childbearing, this slippage of organs can create pressure and discomfort in the lower abdomen. More serious symptoms include disruptive bowel and urinary complications.

The insertion of a pessary—a diaphragm-like device—can help support the uterus. It can be used in combination with an estrogen cream to build up cells, and with pelvic exercises that can strengthen weakened muscles. Over the long term, however, a pessary can cause ulcerations in the vagina. As prolapse becomes more pronounced, a pessary may not be able to support the uterus, and it can interfere with intercourse and provoke incontinence, since it changes the angle of the bladder. A more complete remedy for prolapse involves surgical repair and reconstruction of ligaments and tissues relating to the prolapsed organ. If the removal of the uterus is necessary, it's usually because it has descended too far down the vaginal canal for surgical correction.

Chronic Pelvic Pain

A wide range of disorders can cause chronic pelvic pain. Frequently a specific cause for the pain can be discovered and treated. In some cases, however, the cause remains unknown.

Finding the exact cause of pain often requires a very thorough evaluation. A pelvic exam, laparoscopy, ultrasound examination, and, sometimes if indicated, *magnetic resonance imaging* (MRI) will help establish if the pain is being produced by a gynecologic condition, such as fibroids or endometriosis, or if it is linked to a gastrointestinal, urinary, or muscular cause. Studies have shown that a significant number of chronic pelvic pain cases that reveal no physical problem are associated with a history of childhood sexual abuse. For this reason, many doctors recommend you also seek a psychiatric evaluation to address this issue.

While nonsteroidal anti-inflammatory agents and birth control pills can ease pelvic pain, psychological, nutritional, and other approaches can also help. When no other treatment brings relief, a hysterectomy may serve as a last resort. Unfortunately, even a hysterectomy may not bring relief. One study found that in 22 percent of hysterectomy cases, pain persisted after the operation.

Other Disorders

Drugs are routinely the initial treatment for most gynecological disorders. Yet a hysterectomy can be the first route taken for life-threatening cancerous growth or complications of pregnancy. It may be the only way to eradicate cervical, uterine, or ovarian cancer, or to treat premalignant growth that doesn't respond to other measures. It can also serve as an emergency standby measure during childbirth, should the uterus rupture or excessive hemorrhaging occur.

Removal of the Uterus

In medical terms, a "hysterectomy" or "simple hysterectomy" refers to the removal of just the uterus, or the uterus and attached Fallopian tubes. Physicians remove the uterus either through the vagina *(vaginal hysterectomy)* or through an incision in the abdomen *(abdominal hysterectomy)*. When the uterus is removed vaginally, it's common practice also to remove the cervix, the narrow outer portion of the uterus, because it's difficult to extract the uterus otherwise.

If your uterus is removed, bear in mind that you won't have the telltale signs of irregular bleeding to inform you that you're becoming menopausal. Instead, hot flashes or vaginal dryness may alert you. Since your ovaries are still functioning and your body is still receiving premenopausal amounts of estrogen and other ovarian-made hormones, you will not need to consider hormone replacement after surgery. However, studies indicate that removal of the uterus can hasten the arrival of a natural menopause by an average of four years. The uterus's extraction appears to disrupt blood vessel networks between the uterus and ovaries, resulting in a more rapid depletion of eggs.

If the pear-sized uterus does need to be removed, you well might wonder what takes up its space after it's gone. As it happens, your abdominal cavity is filled with spaces. If it weren't, we'd all be in trouble when our stomach enlarged after a big meal or our bowel expanded. The space left after the uterus is removed isn't very big, and the sur-rounding organs move into it, usually without compromising their existing structure and function.

After this operation, some women report urinary symptoms, constipation, and fatigue, while others report no changes at all. You may experience a decline in sexual responsiveness. According to some studies, as many as 20 to 30 percent of women who have had their uteruses removed have noticed this change. It can be due to the loss of sexual stimulation formerly provided by an intact uterus and cervix. Women who are aware that the cervix's motion can add to the ability to have an orgasm often request an abdominal instead of a vaginal hysterectomy, since the former leaves the cervix in place.

> "I feel exactly the same way I did before my uterus was taken out. It's as if someone took it without my knowing, and the only way I know is by looking down and seeing a six-inch scar. Everything about sex is the same, too."

In a large number of cases, it's also true that a hysterectomy can significantly improve sexual responsiveness and functioning by providing relief from prior symptoms. In general, a hysterectomy can provide such relief from symptoms, many women report feeling better, physically and mentally. If depression results from this operation, usually it's transient. When women are more deeply depressed, their depression often is linked to a chronic pattern of depression.

Removal of the Ovaries

In some 5 to 17 percent of surgeries to remove the uterus, the ovaries are removed at the same time. Such combined surgery—called *hysterectomy with bilateral oophorectomy*—can be necessary if the same condition, such as a malignancy, afflicts both uterus and ovaries. In some cases of endometriosis, the ovaries are also removed, because ovarian hormones can prolong the condition.

If a disorder is severe enough to justify removal of the ovaries, often it has already impinged upon the uterus. If it hasn't, in some cases the removal of the uterus is viewed as a precautionary measure against recurrence. However, when the ovaries are removed for a benign condition, a woman may want to retain her uterus. This way, through egg or embryo donation, she may still be able to experience pregnancy and childbirth.

> "When I was 30, I was out running and started getting really sharp pains in my lower abdomen. It turned out that large cysts had penetrated both ovaries. The left ovary and 90 percent of the right one were removed right away. Prior to all this, I hadn't seen a gynecologist in years. I exercised a lot, so I thought I was in great shape. If I'd gone to the gynecologist, the cyst problem might have been caught early on and I'd still have my ovaries."

A hysterectomy with bilateral oophorectomy may also be recommended for women over 50 who need to have their uterus removed. With the ovaries nearing the end of their egg supply, their removal along with the uterus is often viewed as a preventive strategy against several diseases, particularly ovarian cancer. Although only 1 percent of women develop this cancer within their lifetime, it's difficult to detect or diagnose until far advanced. Even when the ovaries are removed, however, a slight chance of ovarian-like cancer remains.

If you're postmenopausal and have your ovaries re-

A survivor of ovarian cancer recounts, "If you're having your uterus and ovaries removed, as I did, because of a precancerous condition, or a cancerous condition, I strongly recommend an abdominal hysterectomy over a vaginal one. If they remove organs vaginally, they don't have a clear viewing and potentially can miss something. In my case, in 1981 they missed a cancerous tab on the Fallopian tube. Even though my ovaries were gone, ovarian cancer developed over the next several years without my knowing. In 1989 I was operated on abdominally to remove the cancer. I'd had Pap smears all through the '80s. But Pap smears don't pick up ovarian cancer. The symptoms show more through digestion—a lot of gas and finally throwing up."

moved, don't be surprised if you experience hot flashes on the heels of this surgery. You might think that since you've already gone through menopause, you're through with hot flashes. However, recall that your postmenopausal ovaries were still making androgen, some of which got converted to estrogen. This is why removal of the ovaries can prompt a decline in estrogen, which sets off hot flashes.

If a woman age 50 or older has her uterus removed, with her ovaries left intact, there's as much as a 10 percent chance she'll need ovarian surgery in the future because of any one of several disorders. For this reason, a woman age 50 or over who has her uterus removed will often lose her ovaries too. Considering that 90 percent of women will *not* have future problems with their ovaries, a woman this age may want to rethink this common approach. Her ovaries aren't necessarily so expendable, as previously believed. The postmenopausal ovaries continue producing androgen, some of which converts to estrogen and is an important source of a woman's remaining estrogen supply.

Ovarian androgen also may be contributing to a woman's sex drive.

If you're under age 40 and your uterus must be removed, make sure there's a concerted effort to retain your ovaries—unless of course a very serious condition such as cancerous growth or extreme infection precludes this. If you're between the ages of 40 and 50 and must have your uterus removed, the decision to also remove your ovaries should depend on your medical profile, not the 10 percent chance that you may require surgery to remove them in the future. Discuss all your options thoroughly with your doctor and make clear your preference to retain your ovaries if possible. The decision is yours to make after you have all the facts.

If both your ovaries are removed during the premenopausal years, with or without the uterus, menopause will immediately ensue. "Surgical menopause," as it's called, causes a more dramatic drop in estrogen than if menopause arrived naturally and gradually. Hence, your hot flashes may be all the more acute. Surgical menopause deprives women of their main estrogen source months or years ahead of a natural menopause. Consequently, the risk for heart disease and osteoporosis increases, although more for some women than others. As discussed in Sections Two and Three, a variety of treatments and regimes can help compensate for the estrogen loss. The earlier surgical menopause occurs, the more aggressively a woman may want to subscribe to supplemental treatment for bone, heart, and other estrogen-receptive cells.

Removal of your ovaries and uterus/cervix can cause more sexual dysfunction than if only the uterus/cervix is extracted. This is because the estrogen depletion that occurs with the ovaries' loss can contribute to vaginal dryness and other symptoms that may interfere with sexual

"Right after my ovaries were removed, water from night sweats began pouring out of me—literally overnight. When I rolled over, it was like a faucet going on. I was extremely anxious about what was happening to me. I remember thinking that if I had to live like this, I didn't want to. I got no feedback from the doctor. Prior, we had decided I'd go on estrogens to replace what I had lost to surgery. I began taking them, and not long after that my night sweats decreased. But ever since, I've continued to experience occasional night sweats."

activity. Moreover, with the ovaries gone, the decline in androgen levels also appear to prompt a drop in libido, or sexual desire, in some women. Yet human sexuality is a product of more than just pelvic organs and hormones. Many other factors will affect your sex life after hysterectomy, including your beliefs, attitudes, and self-image, as well as those of your partner.

Certain conditions call for the removal of only one ovary. An ovary besieged by a large benign tumor or cysts, for example, might need to be removed. If you have one ovary surgically removed, with or without the uterus, your remaining ovary usually continues releasing enough estrogen to maintain normal periods and keep you headed toward a natural menopause. Generally, supplemental therapy for estrogen and androgen loss shouldn't be necessary.

Other Medical Interventions Connected to an Early Menopause

Sometimes physicians must resort to using chemotherapy or radiation treatment to thwart cancerous growth. Although the ovaries themselves might be disease-free, they can get caught in the line of fire, so to speak, and become the target of potent doses of chemotherapy or radiation. This can cause an irreversible ovarian failure with immediate menopause following. Whenever possible, physicians strive to conserve and protect the ovaries. But necessary treatment for a life-threatening illness will always take first priority.

Chemotherapy

"Many of the most effective drugs used in chemotherapy for cancer unfortunately also can cause infertility," notes Dr. Annekathryn Goodman, MGH gynecologic oncologist.

When circulating in the body, anticancer chemotherapy is designed to kill fast-growing cells, such as those found in malignant tumors. An unintended side effect is the simultaneous destruction of all other types of rapidly dividing tissue, such as hair follicle cells, as well as sperm-producing cells in the male and egg cells in the female. However, while hair loss is reversible after chemotherapy ends, egg loss may be permanent, since a women is born with all the eggs she'll ever have. If egg damage occurs, a drug-induced menopause may ensue.

Chemotherapy's damaging effect isn't an issue for postmenopausal women whose ovarian function has already lapsed. But it can be a very traumatic issue for premenopausal women. For example, when chemotherapy is required for breast cancer, most premenopausal women will lose the function of their ovaries, according to Goodman. However, studies have demonstrated that there's a good chance that chemotherapy won't damage the ovaries of a young woman who hasn't reached puberty.

After puberty, the older the premenopausal woman, the

more susceptible her declining reserve of eggs is to chemotherapy. Among several categories of chemotherapy drugs, alkylating agents are the most potent, especially in higher doses. Alkylating agents linked to infertility include cyclophosphamide, chlorambucil, the mustards, busulfan and procarbazine.

For many women chemotherapy's cruelest blow is its potential for destroying the possibility of future natural pregnancies. A woman can take some comfort in knowing that an expanding range of alternative reproductive approaches is available. Meanwhile, researchers are exploring techniques that might one day protect the ovaries from chemotherapy's harmful effects. In addition, it would be helpful if a successful technique for freezing eggs for future use could be developed. (It does exist for sperm.)

Radiation Treatment

Like chemotherapy, radiation treatment (as opposed to radiation for diagnostic purposes) is used primarily to arrest cancer. Ovarian failure can result if a woman receives large doses of radiation for cancerous growths in or around the pelvis. Such cancers include cervical cancer, sarcoma of the pelvic bones, and lymphoma that involves the pelvic lymph nodes. In some situations, however, surgeons can reposition the ovaries to either side, out of the field of radiation ("ovarian transposition"), to avoid damaging them.

Radiation used for diagnostic X rays—several thousand times less intense than treatment doses—doesn't destroy ovarian cells. However, because there's a concern that diagnostic X rays to the pelvis might alter the genetic material in the ovaries, radiologists try to avoid X rays to the lower abdomen unless medically indicated. When conducting an upper GI series or a chest X ray, just to be on the safe side, health professionals have women wear lead aprons to protect other radiation-sensitive organs, such as the breasts and the thyroid. Generally, physicians try to ensure that pregnant women do not receive X rays. Yet in cases where a pregnancy hasn't yet been detected, and a pregnant woman is X-rayed by mistake, no adverse outcomes have been reported.

If you experience menopause following chemotherapy or radiation therapy, you'll be losing your major source of estrogen at an earlier-than-normal age. You should be especially attentive to your risks of osteoporosis and heart disease. You may need medical, dietary, or other intervention in order to supplement the estrogen that remains in your body.

Medication That Produces Pseudomenopause

As described earlier in this chapter, synthetic drugs called GnRH agonists are frequently used to treat a range of gynecological disorders. This is because of their ability to halt the ovaries' production of estrogen and progesterone by first stopping the pituitary's release of luteinizing hormone (LH). If you suffer from estrogen-fed fibroids, uterine bleeding, or endometriosis, though expensive, these drugs may save you from surgery.

Your menstrual cycle will cease soon after you take GnRH agonists. But this "pseudomenopause" is fully reversible. A few months after you stop taking GnRH agonists, your periods will resume.

3

What Are the Symptoms of Menopause?

While you may think that menopause is heralded by a very specific list of symptoms, a look at different cultural groups around the world reveals that the list is far from universal. Hot flashes and vaginal dryness are the most commonly cited menopausal symptoms in the United States, whereas menopausal women in Java are more apt to complain of fatigue and weight gain. And although American women face a significant increase in the risk for heart disease in the years following menopause, Japanese women encounter a much lower risk. Cultural as well as environmental differences between societies apparently result in very different menopausal outcomes.

In fact, recent research suggests that rather than evaluate menopause as a universal experience, we should try to identify each woman's individual vulnerability to a wide range of possible postmenopausal symptoms and conditions. Your personal susceptibility might depend on your present health, diet, psychological and genetic makeup, and ethnic and/or socioeconomic background.

Any discussion of menopausal changes is confounded by a very large question still beyond our grasp: Which changes are related to menopause itself, and which are part of the aging process? Of course, menopause is itself a component of aging. Yet ovarian failure can trigger certain physical changes that happen irrespective of physical age. For instance, if young female athletes exercise too much, their hypothalamus can close down, blocking the production of ovarian hormones. This can lead to a "pseudo-menopausal" condition: loss of bone density. And yet such women aren't even middle-aged!

Women are apt to blame "the change" for every noticeable twinge or discomfort—headaches, sleeplessness, wrinkling skin, dull or thinning hair, depression, weight gain, decreased muscle tone, lethargy, lack of libido. "Menopause has given me agoraphobia!" claimed one woman. While some of these complaints may be menopause-related, in many cases it remains unclear which symptoms are caused by menopause and which by aging. Moreover, symptoms seemingly tied to menopause may be linked instead to the daily stresses women frequently encounter in midlife. Physical changes can also be caused by a poor diet or an unidentified illness.

Nonetheless, as accumulating evidence keeps showing, a woman's midlife estrogen decline does seem the primary instigator of certain specific symptoms and systemic changes. Considering the myriad types of cells that take in estrogen, it's understandable how estrogen's decline can have a marked effect on everything from bone to heart to brain. Less obvious and less well studied are the effects of reduced levels of progesterone and androgen on post-

menopausal women. Premenopausally, the monthly production of progesterone protects against endometrial cancer and helps to maintain bone. Androgen, research has
revealed, can help supplement bone growth and is thought
to influence sex drive. Yet, more research is needed to better understand the tasks of these hormones and to what
extent menopause alters their effects.

The following discussion of symptoms and systemic
changes is drawn from research primarily involving
women from Western societies and doesn't necessarily reflect how women in other parts of the world experience
menopause.

Irregular Menstrual Bleeding

If you're in your forties or fifties, shorter or longer periods, heavier or lighter menstrual bleeding, and varying
lengths of time between menstrual cycles may be a sign
that perimenopause has begun and menopause is nearing.
You may sometimes experience excessive menstrual-flow
clotting because of irregular ovulation.

A woman age 47 recounts: "Starting about two years ago my
periods started coming every three weeks or so. Just recently
something even more bizarre occurred. I got my period for
two days. Then, right after it stopped, I began getting unmis-
takable signs of PMS—water retention, breast tenderness,
mood swings. Soon after, I got my period again and it lasted
for nine days! I'm healthy otherwise, and my doctor and I
have chalked this up to perimenopausal vacillations."

Keep in mind, however, that for many women your age,
erratic bleeding isn't necessarily a sign of an encroaching

menopause. Instead, it may indicate a gynecologic or other health disorder. Many disorders can present themselves through irregular menstrual flow, including thyroid disorders (hypo- or hyperthyroidism, too little or too much thyroid gland activity respectively) and uterine conditions such as fibroids, polyps, cancerous growths, and hormonal abnormalities. If you're concurrently experiencing any pain and discomfort, urinary or bowel changes, loss of energy or other unusual symptoms, see your health care provider promptly. Irregular menstrual bleeding during perimenopause can be disruptive and annoying, and may include heavy bleeding, clots, and severe cramps, but it shouldn't produce atypical symptoms or unusual pain.

Hot Flashes

If you're experiencing the "classic" symptom of menopause known as the "hot flash," you're hardly alone; approximately 75 percent of women report the same sensation, with 15 to 25 percent severely affected.

This sudden wave of heat typically starts in your torso and neck and spreads upward to your face and down your arms and back. Soon after, you might find that you perspire profusely, then suddenly become chilly. While hot flashes often descend out of the blue, they can be set off by exercise, smoking, alcohol, stress, a hot day, or another source of excess heat. Women are more prone to flashes (and accompanying night sweats) at night. It could be because blankets and bed coverings create more heat, although some women wake up to find themselves soaking wet without even a blanket. Women occasionally report that just before a hot flash occurs, they sense an aura or premonition that it's coming.

"You start sweating as if you'd been really running and don't know why."

"My hot flashes start in my head. My whole head, face, and neck get terribly hot, and then I start sweating. My hot flashes always occur at night."

"Before menopause I experienced terrible night sweats. I'd wake up four to five times in the wee hours of the morning and just be drenched. I'd take the covers off, then get chilly and pull them back up. My legs and boobs would stick together. It was the most uncomfortable feeling I've ever experienced. The sweats especially occurred the week before my period. During the day I'd be a wreck because of lack of sleep. I'd only have one good week a month. Interestingly enough, my mother also had a history of bad night sweats."

While hot flashes aren't painful, they can be very uncomfortable, disruptive, and even embarrassing if they erupt full force at the wrong moment. They can lead to sleeplessness and fatigue, irritability, poor concentration, and forgetfulness. As for poor sleep quality, no evidence ties wakeful nights directly to ovarian failure. If that were true, postmenopausal women might never again get a good night's sleep. It appears to be hot flashes—which can awaken a woman, or come and go as she sleeps—that can interrupt sleep, sometimes resulting in drenching night sweats.

Usually starting in the perimenopausal years, hot flashes can show up before any noticeable changes occur in your menstrual pattern. Not infrequently, they persist past menopause, although studies have shown that they often fade away after the last menstrual cycle. On the other hand, some women don't experience the symptom until after menopause.

On average, menopausal hot flashes last from six months to three years. Eighty percent of women who experience hot flashes have them for at least one year, with 25 percent of women riding them out for over five years. Occasionally the symptom still manifests itself in 70- and 80-year-old women. The frequency of hot flashes runs the gamut. They can occur every few minutes, every few hours, once a week, once a month, or even for just one fleeting moment in a woman's life. An episode might last for a few seconds or a few minutes.

> A 51-year-old woman recounts, "I still get my periods, and I've had hot flashes for about five years. They especially happen when I'm anxious, and the worst part was that they used to make my glasses fog up. At work, I'd be talking to someone in upper management, and they'd just fog up. It was totally embarrassing. My eye doctor recommended new glasses—the bottom of the frame is lifted off my cheeks—and thank heavens it solved the problem. But the hot flashes continue and I get so red in the face. And I never was a blusher!"

Researchers in the 1980s theorized that a hot flash, known medically as *vasomotor flushing,* is a direct response to a menopausal drop in estrogen. Women who are born with ovaries that lack the ability to produce eggs and estrogen, a condition seen in patients with Turner's syndrome, provide an important clue to estrogen's role. Normally such women experience no menstruation, no menopause, no hot flashes. Yet when they go on estrogen therapy and subsequently go off it, they have hot flashes. Another clue that strongly implies the estrogen–hot flash connection is that estrogen therapy is 95 percent effective in treating hot flashes. Flashes appear linked to the actual *decline* in estrogen, not its low levels. If the latter were true, women would be getting hot flashes for the rest of their lives.

> "So many of my friends get night sweats, but I just get hot flashes during the day. No night sweats. Once I got hot flashes and hives combined!"

The exact mechanisms that produce a hot flash as estrogen declines are still under investigation. One theory proposes that as estradiol levels diminish, neurotransmitters in the brain are thrown out of balance. This alteration of brain chemistry appears in turn to cause a sudden drop in the body's internal thermostat, located in the hypothalamus. Receiving the message to cool down, the body rushes blood from the liver, the heart, and other warmer "core" areas to the skin for cooling. Thus, internal heat is transferred to the extremities. Peripheral (away from the center of the body) blood vessels widen, the heart rate accelerates, and skin temperature rises as much as 10° to 15° degrees Fahrenheit. Sweating then occurs to cool the body through water evaporation. When the hypothalamus's temperature gauge returns to normal, the body feels all the chillier because of the heat just released. To warm up the core again, peripheral blood vessels constrict to return blood from the extremities, and shivering begins—muscle contractions that produce heat. The term "vasomotor flushing" appropriately refers to the nerves and muscles that are dilating and constricting the blood vessels as a hot flash cycles.

Generally, overweight women report milder hot flashes than thinner women. This appears to be because they undergo less of an estrogen decline, since they have more peripheral fat cells that convert androgens into estrogens. Smokers, meanwhile, may undergo more intense flashes. Researchers believe this is because a smoker converts fewer androgens to estrogens, reducing overall circulating estrogen and making the decline in estrogen all the more pronounced. (Hence, smokers may be at greater risk for osteoporosis.)

> "Do you know why cardigans were invented as opposed to pullovers? So you can rip them off quickly when you're having a hot flash!"

For a woman facing ovarian failure caused by surgery or other medical intervention, an abrupt drop in estrogen can instigate acute hot flashes while she's still in the recovery room. A postmenopausal woman who has her ovaries removed also may experience hot flashes. This is because postmenopausal ovaries still make considerable amounts of androgen, some of which converts to estrogen. Therefore removal of postmenopausal ovaries can precipitate some decline in estrogen.

In unpublished data stemming from the Massachusetts Women's Health Study, 19 percent of postmenopausal women reported never having experienced hot flashes. For many others, hot flashes remain minor inconveniences. All in all, women should realize that most cases of hot flashes are easily surmountable. Even the most severe cases are 95 percent treatable. Some women regard them as emblematic of what anthropologist Margaret Mead referred to as "postmenopausal zest." As one bumper sticker reads, I DON'T GET HOT FLASHES, I GET POWER SURGES.

Vaginal and Urinary Tract Changes

A woman's genital and urinary organs are made up of tissues that are "target-specific" for estrogen circulating in the blood, and estrogen plays a significant role in maintaining their cellular structure and function. Hence, when estrogen declines upon menopause, the vagina, vulva, bladder, urethra, and uterus are all the more susceptible to atrophy or deterioration. Since aging further influences urogenital atrophy, postmenopausal women are more prone to a range of associated urinary tract and genital disorders than they were before.

Urinary tract atrophy, perpetuated by both estrogen loss and aging, can contribute to incontinence, or the involuntary leakage of urine; infection; painful urination *(dysuria)*; itching *(pruritus)*; and urinary frequency, urgency, and other urinary tract problems. One of the most common symptoms associated with vaginal atrophy is vaginal dryness, although vaginal itching, irritation, and inflammation can also result from estrogen decline and age.

> "It wasn't long after having two babies that I began urinating more and more frequently. The older I got, the less I could hold, the more often I had to go. It got to the point where I had to urinate every fifteen or twenty minutes. If I went out with friends, I never drank fluids. When I went anywhere, I had to plan my outings around bathrooms. Where was the bathroom in the mall? Could I drive from point A to point B without having to stop?"

With aging, some women experience prolapse of the bladder or uterus. Prolapse refers to an organ's slipping out of its normal position. Its primary cause is an age-related weakening of an organ's supporting ligaments. However, weakened tissue can be further exacerbated by estrogen depletion.

Vaginal Dryness

As soon as one to three months after menopause, the vagina can show the effects of estrogen depletion. As the vaginal lining thins, the normal folds of tissue *(rugae)* flatten out inside the vagina, and the underlying blood vessels narrow. In time the whole vagina shortens, much the way the uterus shrinks when estrogen is withdrawn. With estrogen no longer stimulating vaginal secretants, the vagina becomes dryer and less self-lubricated. Add in the factors that estrogen reduction can also lead to the constriction of the vaginal opening and decrease glandular lubrication at the time of intercourse, and it's not surprising that some postmenopausal women find intercourse uncomfortable, even painful.

> "Within six years after menopause I had no interest in sex with my husband anymore—because it felt like I was having sex with razor blades. No kidding, the dryness was that bad."

Though only a small percentage of women complain of vaginal dryness in the years immediately following menopause, gynecologists have observed that the problem is progressive and can become considerably more pronounced within ten years. Some gynecologists estimate that at least 50 percent of women over age 60 show some degree of vaginal dryness. In the most noticeable cases, vaginal dryness produces chafing and irritation of the labia, as well as painful intercourse. Yet a decrease in vaginal lubrication doesn't become problematic for many women, since some lubrication may still be derived from both the estrogen remaining in the body and from the Bartholin's glands, small glands located at the entrance of the vagina. The stimulation of sex itself, it's long been noted, can help keep the postmenopausal vagina lubricated and toned.

Vaginal and Urinary Tract Infection (UTI)

When menopause diminishes your estrogen supply, the acidic vaginal environment may also decline, as can a variety of beneficial natural bacteria that facilitate acidic conditions. This creates a more favorable environment for other bacteria that can cause vaginal infections and resulting discharge. However, the opportunity for infection varies greatly among postmenopausal women. In some, enough natural bacteria still flourish to protect against undesirable intruders. Other women have no beneficial microbes and are plagued with recurrent infections.

Gynecologists theorize that lower estrogen levels after menopause may similarly contribute to urinary tract infections (UTIs). Infections of the vagina and urinary system can sometimes be interrelated. As acidic levels in the vagina change to more alkaline states and detrimental bacteria colonize the vagina, they may subsequently spread to the bladder, causing infection. Also, as some women age, their urine becomes less acidic, hence more vulnerable to disease-bearing bacteria. It's unknown if this is due to estrogen loss or aging. Finally, the thinning of the urethra may result in more UTIs.

Urinary Incontinence

Urinary incontinence, or the inability to control urine flow, affects 15 to 35 percent of women over the age of 60, according to recent reports. (This figure doesn't include women in nursing homes, where the incidence rate is much greater.) Other sources suggest an even higher frequency, since many women are reluctant to talk to their physician about incontinence.

Gynecologists note a definite rise in incontinence among women after menopause. While the condition increasingly shows up in later life, it's not unusual for women to begin experiencing it one to two years after menopause.

Although researchers generally agree that estrogen depletion usually isn't the root cause of incontinence, it can exacerbate the condition. In cases in which aging may already have lessened pelvic floor muscle strength and altered bladder and urinary tract function, estrogen loss can further augment the aging effects that contribute to incontinence. In order for the bladder to store urine and empty in a coordinated fashion into the *urethra* (the tube that runs from the bladder to the external surface), the urethra needs to retain a certain tightness or resistance. Loss of estrogen appears to relax the urethra's structure, contributing to incontinence.

Incontinence in both women and men generally can be divided into two different types. In *urge incontinence,* a strong desire to void (urgency) is followed by unstoppable urine loss. The cause of urge incontinence is often linked to an overactive detrusor muscle in the bladder wall, which is responsible for contracting the bladder.

With *stress incontinence,* you may not feel the urge to go, but sudden increases in abdominal pressure can result in involuntary urine loss. Stress incontinence is usually provoked by physical activity; coughing, sneezing, laughing, jogging, aerobic exercise, squash, and other sports can produce leakage. It occurs because sudden increases in abdominal pressure compress the bladder and exceed the resisting backflow pressure of the urethra. The urethra acts as a sphincter (much like a washer in a faucet), and any weakness in the position of the urethra and bladder neck can undermine this mechanism. A poorly supported bladder neck, perhaps weakened by pregnancy and childbirth as well as estrogen depletion and aging, permits more pressure on the bladder and less on the bladder outlet. In many cases of stress incontinence, the pelvic floor, which normally helps support the bladder neck, has dropped, allowing urine to leak out when there's pressure on the bladder.

> "Because of stress incontinence, if I sneezed, coughed, or laughed, I'd lose my urine. When I lifted my leg to step up on a curb, I'd lose urine. They discovered I had a dropped bladder."

Other Urogenital Disorders

The depletion of estrogen and associated physiological changes, such as decreased blood flow, decreased muscle tone, and slowed tissue growth, can cause inflammation of the vagina *(vaginitis)*, especially if your vagina is dry when you have intercourse. Lowered estrogen levels can also contribute to atrophy of the urethra and other urinary tract features that can result in inflammation of the urethra *(urethritis)*, painful urination *(dysuria)*, the frequent need to urinate (frequency), the urge to urinate even if the bladder isn't full (urgency), and inflammation of the bladder *(cystitis)*.

In cases of postmenopausal urogenital prolapse, gynecologists usually regard estrogen depletion as only one of several promoting factors. Age and other circumstances play a role, as is true for all the urogenital disorders described above.

Skin

By your forties and fifties, your skin starts showing the effects of cumulative exposure to the sun's ultraviolet light and the toll of advancing years. Smoking can also further damage the skin by restricting blood flow to the skin's supporting layers.

"The great majority of what we perceive as aging of the skin—such as wrinkling, sun freckles, age marks, mottling of pigmentation, and broken blood vessels—is actually due to the sun," observes Dr. Elaine Kaye, a dermatologist at MGH. With time, skin becomes dryer, less elastic, and more prone to wrinkling. Research is showing that menopause's withdrawal of hormones may also deal a blow to the *dermis,* the layer of skin below the *epidermis,* the outer layer. Menopause may contribute to the thinning of your skin, making it all the more vulnerable to sun and time.

Both estrogen and androgen apparently play a part in maintaining the dermis, since receptors for both are lodged in the dermis's connective tissue. Some studies show that estrogen has the ability to both add to the thickness of skin and augment its content of collagen, the protein that builds the fibrous base of all connective tissue, including skin and bone. Estrogen is thought to increase the production of collagen while replenishing the fluid content between connective-tissue cells. Androgen appears to stimulate skin thickness, by stimulating proliferation of cells in the dermis.

Since both skin and bone are forms of connective tissue supported by collagen, they share a similar vulnerability to estrogen depletion. Similar to bone loss after menopause, the loss of skin collagen happens at a faster rate in the early postmenopausal years than in later years. Studies show some 30 percent of skin collagen is lost in the first five years. In comparison, skin thickness, although closely associated with skin collagen, appears to decrease more gradually.

Some women report that after menopause their skin becomes that much more susceptible to surface changes: bruising and age marks, flaking and mottling. Further investigation is needed in this area before anyone can say with any certainty if menopause, as opposed to aging, leads to skin's decline.

Hair

When estrogen levels fall after menopause, the increased proportion of male hormones to female hormones in a postmenopausal woman's system can cause her to develop more facial hair, particularly on the upper lip and chin.

Some women experience progressive thinning of their hair after menopause, although the two events aren't necessarily related. However, some women do exhibit hair loss as a result of similar hormonal shifts related to childbearing, ovarian failure, and other endocrine-connected events. It's still less than clear, however, how much menopause contributes to changes in scalp hair, including growth rate, texture, or graying. With aging, there is a decrease in pubic hair.

Indigestion and Constipation

While some women mention increasing problems with digestion and constipation beginning soon after menopause, mainstream medicine has left these complaints largely unexplored. However, practicioners of alternative medicine frequently report treating intestinal disorders in women in their postmenopausal years.

"Menopausal constipation and indigestion are generally due to the slowing of the gastrointestinal tract (estrogen is a gastrointestinal stimulant) and heavy demands on the liver," writes Susun S. Weed, herbal consultant and author of *Menopausal Years: The Wise Woman Way*. "When your levels of estrogen and progesterone change . . . your bowel patterns change, too." As valid as such observations might be, medical research has yet to confirm such reports.

Dry-Eye

Dry-eye, a condition that reduces the eye's tear film and leaves eyes itchy and irritated, afflicts an estimated 40 percent of women and men at some point in their lives. Many more women than men are affected by the condition. Among the many different contributors to dry-eye, ophthalmologists and optometrists recognize menopause's hormonal decline as being a frequent, credible cause, although one not broadly researched. Like many other postmenopausal women, you might have overlooked a possible connection between menopause and dry eyes.

"I see women come in here all the time—age 50 and over—complaining of dry-eyedness. They usually don't realize that it can be due to menopausal hormonal changes," notes Dr. Cynthia D'Auria, an optometrist associated with the New England Medical Center and Tufts University School of Medicine in Boston. Postmenopausal contact lens wearers especially complain of dry-eye, since contact lens comfort is dependent upon an adequate tear supply, according to D'Auria.

Because dry-eye also commonly occurs among pregnant women whose estrogen levels are high, some researchers suspect that conditions other than estrogen deficiency may contribute to dry-eye. Low androgen levels may be the culprit, since both postmenopausal and pregnant women have relatively lower levels of this hormone. Researchers holding this view recommend a low-dose androgen supplement to restore normal tear-gland function. Since other recent studies suggest that estrogen therapy can improve tear-film deficiencies, further research is clearly needed to clarify what part estrogen and androgen play in lubricating the eye.

Memory and Brain Functioning

Filled with estrogen receptors, your brain—just like your bone and breast tissue—is exposed to significant amounts of circulating estrogens. Several new studies suggest not only that estrogen plays an appreciable role in brain functioning, notably memory, but also that its decline after menopause may be linked to some types of dementia such as Alzheimer's disease. However, neuroscientists caution that women should not think that once they hit menopause, their gray cells are going to fizzle. The findings are still far too preliminary to draw such conclusions. If they have merit, it's likely that, as in the case of so many other changes tied to estrogen's decline, some women are more susceptible to estrogen-related brain alterations than others. In regard to Alzheimer's, it's worth noting that researchers have linked the disease to inherited genes, with possibly other culprit gene sites yet to be identified. So estrogen's decline is unlikely to be the only factor precipitating Alzheimer's.

Estrogen's influence on the brain is no small matter, for it actually promotes growth in brain cells, specifically in the regions of the *cerebral cortex* and the *hypothalamus*. Researchers have discovered that estrogen also prompts the growth of nerve cell extensions (*axons* and *dendrites*) and supports the communication "links" *(synapses)* between brain nerve cells.

Estrogen's ability to protect brain activity in post-menopausal women receiving estrogen supplements was strongly hinted at in a comprehensive study reported in 1993. Among a group of 2,418 women in a Southern California retirement community, those on estrogen supplements were 40 percent less likely to have Alzheimer's than those who hadn't taken the hormone. Higher estrogen doses were associated with a lower risk for the disease, reported study leader Dr. Victor Henderson of the University of Southern California. However, it's possible that women who choose to take hormones may, to begin with, be in better health. Those studied, therefore, might have been less prone to Alzheimer's whether or not they were on hormone replacement therapy, or HRT.

Alzheimer's seldom strikes younger men and women,

with less than 2 percent of Americans under the age of 55 afflicted. Yet some 50 percent of Americans over age 85 have the disease, and—perhaps because they are more likely to live longer—the majority are women. "There's clear-cut evidence that women are twice as likely to get Alzheimer's then men," according to Dr. Dominique Toran-Allerand, a neuroscientist at Columbia University College of Physicians and Surgeons. Why are women more susceptible to the condition? Some researchers speculate that it's because men, in whom testosterone's conversion to estrogen also appears to protect brain functioning, have the benefit of fairly high testosterone levels throughout their lifetime. Women might more easily fall victim to Alzheimer's because they lose estrogen with menopause, theorize scientists.

Osteoporosis

If there's anything good to be said about osteoporosis, it's that many of you reading this won't experience this debilitating, bone-robbing condition. As many as three-quarters of women are not affected by it. What's striking about this condition, however, is that women account for 80 percent of its reported 25 million victims in this country, according to the National Osteoporosis Foundation.

For both sexes, numerous known factors can accelerate this disorder, which progressively undermines healthy bone tissue and leaves brittle bone in its wake. Dubbed "the silent thief," osteoporosis can work its damage for years unnoticed until a fracture in the hip, wrist, spine, or other bone brings it to light. Women are much more vulnerable to osteoporosis' ravages than men, since menopause's depletion of hormones represents a signifi-

Figure 5. Normal vs. Osteoporotic Bone

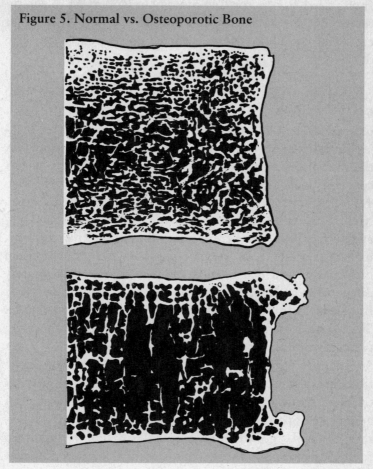

Both these X rays were taken from a thick slice of bone from a vertebra. The normal bone (above) *shows a healthy network of bone tissue (white). The osteoporotic bone* (below) *increases the porosity of the vertebrae and greatly weakens them, raising the risk for spinal fractures.*

Illustration: Harriet Greenfield.

cant added risk factor. Maintains Dr. Robert M. Neer, director of the MGH's Osteoporosis Center, "All other causes of osteoporosis are dwarfed compared to estrogen deficiency."

When you're in your late teens, your bone mineral reaches its peak density and remains at high levels until age 35 to 40. At this point it begins declining at the gradual rate of 1 to 2 percent per year until menopause. Studies reveal that starting in the first year after menopause, the rate of bone-mass loss sharply increases to 2 to 4 percent per year, until the rate slows to approximately 1 to 1.5 percent eight to ten years after menopause. Menopause, therefore, appears to exert an immediate negative effect on bone, a trend that takes its greatest toll during the first five postmenopausal years. Between menopause and death, most women lose approximately 30 percent of their peak bone mass, according to Neer. But bear in mind that these figures reflect the average. Since bone loss rates vary greatly among women, these figures may not reflect your own experience.

How much bone mass you lose due to estrogen depletion can depend on whether you're a fast or a slow loser of bone, your bone density as a young adult, and your age at menopause, notes Neer. Menopause at an earlier-than-normal age—due to surgical ovarian removal or premature ovarian failure—increases the chances of osteoporosis, because the protective effect of estrogen is lost earlier. Younger women who overexercise so much that they lose their periods, and thus their high levels of estrogen, can develop acute signs of osteoporosis. Some endocrinologists claim this is proof that osteoporosis has less to do with aging than with estrogen depletion.

Healthy bone constantly undergoes a process known as

bone remodeling. As old bone gets broken down, new bone replaces it. Osteoporosis begins when the rate of breakdown *(resorption)* exceeds the rate of new bone for-

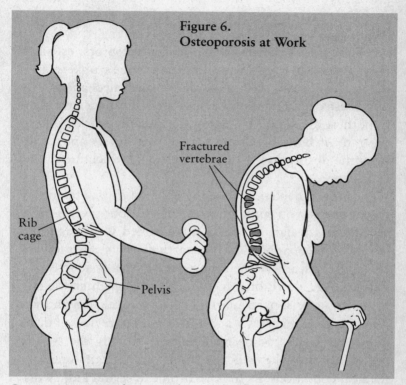

**Figure 6.
Osteoporosis at Work**

Fractured vertebrae

Rib cage

Pelvis

Osteoporosis sets the stage for vertebral fractures, which eventually result in a distortion of the normal spinal curve. The loss of height and stooped carriage may be less troubling than many of the unseen effects of severe osteoporosis. As spinal support declines and the rib cage sinks toward the pelvis, internal organs become cramped, creating breathing difficulties and gastrointestinal discomfort.

Illustration: Harriet Greenfield;
caption: Harvard Medical School Health Publications Group.

mation—a development in later life that becomes as much age-driven as hormone-derived. The frequently used statistic that one-third of women over age 65 have osteoporosis is "off the mark," maintains Neer, who points out that "If a person lives long enough, he or she will get osteoporosis."

Since bone is replete with estrogen receptors, estrogen may directly and indirectly influence bone's upkeep in a number of ways. Although the exact mechanisms by which estrogen retards bone loss are still under investigation, there are signs that estrogen especially works to keep the rate of bone breakdown at normal levels and facilitates the absorption of dietary calcium, which aids bone formation.

If estrogen depletion were the only major risk factor for osteoporosis, you could guard against it. But several other risk factors weigh in. Thin, small-boned Caucasian and Asian women appear to be particularly susceptible to bone loss, as are women who are physically inactive or who smoke. Nutritional factors can also heighten the risk for osteoporosis, particularly diets low in calcium and vitamin D. (See Chapters 9 and 10 for a fuller review of diet's effects on bone.) Some medications, notably the steroid group, can provoke osteoporosis as well, as can numerous medical conditions, including chronic liver and kidney disease, rheumatoid arthritis, an overactive thyroid, and other endocrine disorders.

A susceptibility to osteoporosis can run in the family, through the type of bone structure a person inherits and the inheritance or noninheritance of genetic traits linked to osteoporosis. Bone specialists have had good reason to believe that a risk for osteoporosis can be passed down genetically through generations, and a 1994 Australian study has pinpointed one of the actual genes involved. Researchers at the Garvan Institute of Medical Research in Sydney have identified a gene that is capable of influencing the rate of bone loss due to its regulation of receptors for vitamin D, a key player in bone formation. An exciting finding, this suggests that someday a person might receive a simple blood test that could detect genetic risks for osteoporosis, allowing early treatment.

Although osteoporosis cannot be significantly reversed, treatment for bone loss can slow its pace. (For a discussion of treatments for osteoporosis, see Chapters 6, 9, and 10.)

As more becomes known about osteoporosis, researchers hope that new data will help explain why in some parts of the world osteoporosis seems to be more prevalent today than in years past, a troubling trend suggested by recent studies. In Britain, scientists reported a doubling of hip fractures in both women and men over the last thirty years. Also in Britain, thigh bones from women who died one to two centuries ago were found to be denser and stronger than those of living women. In this country, since records started being kept, the age-specific incidence of fractures has been rising steadily.

Scientists speculate that men and women might have had stronger bones in past eras because they engaged in more physical activity in a more rural environment. In today's world of cars, computers, and cities, our bones simply might not be getting the bone-enhancing exercise our ancestors got. (For exercise's effects on bone, see Chapter 9.)

Heart Disease

The incidence of heart disease in women is considerably low before menopause; after that, it rises. Premenopausally, women face only one-fifth the mortality rate for cardiovascular disease that men face at a comparable age. Yet in the years following menopause, women rapidly become as prone to cardiac mortality as men. For women between the ages of 65 and 70, heart disease becomes the leading cause of death, dwarfing all others. In this age group, cardiovascular disease accounts for over 50 percent of all deaths. In comparison, breast cancer accounts for less than 5 percent.

Does this mean that menopause's withdrawal of estrogen is as harmful to the cardiovascular system as it is to bone? Scientists strongly suspect as much, but absolute proof is still lacking. Nonetheless, certain clues point to a connection between estrogen and heart disease. For instance, women who have their ovaries removed, thus undergoing an earlier-than-natural menopause, have twice the risk for cardiovascular disease than other women their age. Also, research has demonstrated that menopause is associated with a slow rise in low-density lipoprotein (LDL), the so-called "bad" cholesterol. Age-related, LDL lends itself to the formation of *plaque*, blockages in coronary artery blood vessels. Menopause may also precipitate a decrease in high-density lipoprotein (HDL), the "good" lipoprotein that acts like a scavenger to remove bad cholesterol from the bloodstream.

In other words, menopause possibly can contribute to atherosclerosis, especially in women susceptible to this major heart-disease condition. Atherosclerosis happens in this way: As plaque (composed of cholesterol and fats) builds up on the walls of arteries that carry blood and oxygen to the heart, the vessels narrow and less oxygen reaches the heart muscles. A heart attack can ensue if a portion of the heart muscle dies from oxygen deprivation.

If natural estrogen actually works to protect the circulatory system in premenopausal women, just as replacement estrogens appear to do in postmenopausal women—or so the most recent research indicates—estrogen may be functioning to decrease atherosclerosis by inhibiting cholesterol and plaque formation. In general, it may be affecting a range of metabolic, endocrine, and physiological features that help prevent cardiovascular disease, particularly atherosclerosis. Estrogen might work as a vasodilator, widening coronary arteries and adding to their pliability. It may also benefit muscles in vessel walls and the heart itself. While research has clearly documented these effects, deciphering the specific relationship between estrogen and various cardiovascular components remains a goal of further research.

Despite the many telltales that suggest that a woman loses some degree of cardiovascular protection after menopause, many questions await answers. How much cardiovascular decline is due to menopause, how much to aging? What exactly is the rate of decline? One especially perplexing question: When a 30-year-old woman's ovaries are removed and ovarian failure ensues, why is it that the resulting estrogen decline produces no detrimental swing in her cholesterol levels compared with women after menopause? For now, one conceivable explanation is that a 30-year-old woman lacks certain aging factors that, in postmenopausal women, interact with ovarian failure to cause changes in cholesterol. Although her cholesterol might remain unchanged, this 30-year-old woman nevertheless would still be at an increased risk for heart disease because of her lack of ovarian estrogen.

4

New Insights into Menopause and Mood, Sexual Functioning, and Weight

In a 1906 text on the treatment of nervous disorders, a Swiss neuropathologist made the observation that the bad reputation given to mothers-in-law must be attributable to menopause. "In many their character is changed; they become difficult to please and sharp-spoken. . . . It is also the age when one sees the beginning of hypochondriacal and melancholic conditions."

Doom and gloom! How prior generations saddled menopause with a barrage of fearful consequences: deep depression, nervous disorders leading to psychosis, loss of attractiveness, a deadening of sexual desire and ability. Menopause was considered the "dangerous" age, when all this and more could befall a woman. What is often overlooked in retrospective views of women in former times is that menopause often coincided with a range of then-untreatable medical problems. So, indeed, menopause *could* be a dangerous age in that respect.

Rest assured, there is nothing inherently dangerous about menopause itself. Researchers are finding that, in fact, women show no unusually high incidence of depression during menopause and the years immediately following. For a majority of women, the years after this transition may prove to be more depression-free than earlier periods in their lives. Although aging combined with the effects of menopause can contribute to a reduction in sexual functioning as a woman grows older, couples can find sexual fulfillment through many different avenues, and many women report that sexual enjoyment continues straight on into their later years. As for the fear that menopause instantly eviscerates physical attractiveness or mental acuity, you needn't look far—only as far as a relative or a friend—to realize this simply isn't true. No doubt you'd also like to hear that menopause has no bearing on weight gain. Given recent findings, however, there may be some validity in the long-held supposition that menopause can contribute to weight gain and a change in weight distribution.

Taken in total, however, the "change of life" is something of a misnomer. For most of you, especially those in good health, life isn't going to change as drastically or as abruptly as the term "change of life" implies. As baby boomers enter menopause, their collective experience should help reiterate that "the change," overall, isn't a devastating one.

Mood Swings and Depression

Studies are showing that menopause itself doesn't appear to make women prone to depression. However, there's evidence that perimenopause, and its ovarian hormonal decline, may contribute to mood swings and depression in a minority of women. So too can supplemental hormones taken after menopause. In both these cases, mood changes may be caused by changing levels of hormones, which produce alterations in neurotransmitters or brain chemicals.

PMS, or premenstrual syndrome, also seems to result from brain chemical oscillations, according to many researchers. If you've never experienced PMS, probably you have friends who have. The classic signs of PMS—anxiety, depression, and mood turns—are felt to some degree by 15 to 30 percent of women, usually during the days leading up to a period. It's thought that the higher levels of progesterone that circulate after ovulation influence a decline in the levels of serotonin, endorphins, and possibly other brain chemicals. Supporting this theory is the finding that women who don't ovulate, and therefore don't produce progesterone, don't get PMS. Women are most prone to PMS when progesterone is most active. They report feeling their best when rising levels of estrogen are unopposed by progesterone. This happens right before ovulation—that is, before a menstrual cycle's midpoint. Women who have severe PMS are not more likely to have perimenopausal depression.

Mood and Perimenopause

Along with premenstrual and postnatal depression, the years just before menopause appear to mark a peak period for depression in women, recent studies suggest. As reported in the journal *Menopause* by Drs. John W. W. Studd and Roger N. J. Smith of the Chelsea and Westminster Hospital in London, England:

A study by Bungay et. al. "found a clear peak in psychological symptoms and insomnia in women but not men between 45 and 50 years, which preceded by five years the peak incidence of hot flashes and sweats. This suggests that symptoms of depression are not simply a secondary effect of hot flashes, night sweats, and insomnia. Furthermore, this peak incidence of psychological symptoms coincides with the greatest rate of decline of estradiol levels, which usually occurs several years before periods stop."

Since men don't seem to exhibit this pre-midlife slump, there's all the more reason to believe that waning ovarian hormones are playing a role.

It must be emphasized, however, that even if perimenopause does constitute a susceptibility to depression among women (and some studies oppose this finding), only a minority is affected. Moreover, a middle-aged woman's life may be filled with many other factors that might be influencing mood: career pressures, marriage pressures, the care of children or aging parents, to name a few. At any given time, regardless of menopausal status, a reported 10 percent of women show signs of depression. Overall, women are twice as susceptible to depression and related disorders as men. Again, this finding is not necessarily tied to fluctuating hormones.

If the perimenopausal years represent a sinkhole for depression in some women, some researchers speculate that it's because gradually declining levels of estrogen are changing serotonin and other neurotransmitter activity. Just as the *decline* of estrogen, rather than its low levels, is

"Before menopause, my sense of well-being plummeted. It wasn't exactly depression, but I felt I had aged. I also felt as if I was drying up. My breasts had shrunk, and I just felt old."

thought to kindle hot flashes, Studd and Smith theorize that estrogen's downward fall may be the triggering factor. "Once the menopause has been successfully traversed and hormone levels, although low, are once more stable there appears to be no excess of depression in women," the physicians reported in *Menopause*.

> "The same year I turned 50 my son turned 16. What with the mood swings I was going through just before menopause and my son going through teenage-adolescence, I thought we were going to kill each other."

Some researchers question the heavy emphasis put on fluctuating hormone levels and mood. By putting the blame on hormones, they contend, we may not be paying enough attention to other aspects of a woman's life that could be causing depression.

During perimenopause and early postmenopause, hot flashes and night sweats wake some women throughout the night. This can cause chronic sleeplessness, which in turn can exacerbate depression, not to mention irritability, tension, lethargy, and poor concentration. The Massachusetts Women's Health Study found a higher rate of depression in women whose perimenopause lasted longer than twenty-seven months, as compared to those who experienced a shorter perimenopause. If you find yourself waking often because of menopausal symptoms, discuss it with your doctor.

Mood and Menopause

Tracking hundreds of women passing through menopause, two long-term studies have helped quell the myth that menopause can "thoroughly unhinge" women, as one nineteenth-century practitioner put it. Data from the Massachusetts Women's Health Study and a survey led by Karen A. Matthews, a University of Pittsburgh psychologist, found no link between menopause and depression. Both studies also noted that women who approached the transition with more negative expectations often wound up being the most affected by it, emotionally and physically. Comparatively, women who approach menopause without any qualms seem to traverse it with fewer complaints and symptoms. As mentioned in the Introduction, a positive or negative anticipation of menopause may be rooted in a society's overall acceptance or disparagement of this passage point, and in that society's level of respect for older women.

As for the minority of women who become depressed upon menopause, "They're apt to have been depressed prior to menopause," says Nancy E. Avis, a psychologist at the New England Research Institutes and coauthor of the Massachusetts study. When a woman becomes depressed during or following menopause, it may be linked to an ongoing syndrome or a family history of depression. Depression is also often tied to any one of numerous stressful circumstances that women frequently encounter in the adult years, especially midlife—the illness or death of a parent, an individual's own health or sense of aging, career demands or a career change, financial strains, marriage or singleness, or the "empty nest syndrome" (children having left home). What can't be ignored is that for women the rate of death from suicide is highest during midlife (ages 45 to 54) than at any other period in their lives. But there's no evidence that this is due to lowered hormone levels. Boston University gerontologist Elizabeth

W. Markson maintains that the high suicide rate shows instead that midlife can be an exceptionally difficult time for those who are depressed to begin with, and that a greater number of depressed women at this age are apt to contemplate suicide.

Along with the hot flashes and night sweats that may last into the postmenopausal years, vaginal dryness can indirectly lend to anxiety, even depression. In gynecological literature, reports describe postmenopausal women who, having been sexually active before menopause, start withdrawing from sex because of painful intercourse. Depression and even marital difficulties can arise if a woman and her partner fail to recognize vaginal dryness as the problem and instead begin questioning their own or their partner's ability to be sexually aroused.

Mood and Surgical Menopause

The only time when menopause (and not its symptoms) appears to directly give rise to depression is when it is artificially induced through the removal of the ovaries or the removal of the ovaries, uterus, and cervix. Yet, again, only a minority of women are so affected. For many others, a surgical menopause instead provides relief from a disabling or painful disorder. As reported by the Massachusetts Women's Health Study, nearly 50 percent of women who had undergone a surgical menopause reported relief.

Depression related to a *bilateral oophorectomy*—removal of both ovaries—is believed to stem from the abrupt withdrawal of ovarian estrogens. In most cases, it is reported to be transitory and not long-lasting, which fits with the theory that as estrogen levels—even low levels—stabilize, so does mood. When both ovaries are removed, some women report a diminished libido, which researchers believe can result from lowered ovarian androgen. A flagging libido also can contribute to depression, as can the diminished sexual stimulation experienced by some women after the removal of the uterus and cervix.

Mood and Hormone Replacement Therapy (HRT)

The standard hormone replacement prescription for postmenopausal women combines supplemental estrogens with progestins. (A full explanation of HRT occurs in the next chapter.) Progestins are usually an obligatory part of HRT for women with an intact uterus, since they safeguard against endometrial cancer. However, just as natural estrogen and progestin cycling in the body are believed to aggravate PMS, progestin supplements also can produce PMS-like symptoms: mood swings, breast tenderness, irritability, and "the blues." The more susceptible a woman was to PMS before menopause, the greater the chance she'll experience these HRT-induced side effects.

When a woman is just starting on HRT, and doses aren't yet "tailor-made" for her system, progestin-caused mood fluctuations and anxiety can be especially troublesome. Lowering the progestin dosage often returns a woman to normal. Changing from oral (pill form) progestins to nonoral routes, such as injected progestins or progesterone suppositories, can relieve PMS-like symptoms in a small minority of patients. More studies are awaited that can further confirm this. If side effects prove particularly bothersome, progestins may need to be halted. (For a fuller discussion of estrogens taken alone, as well as combined estrogen-progestin therapy, see Chapter 7.)

Menopause and Sexual Functioning

Years ago, there were those that believed that menopause marked the end of a woman's sex life. Thankfully, this myth has been laid to rest. It's true, however, that post-menopausal physical changes can lead to a gradual decline in sexual activity as a woman ages, albeit more in some women than others. Before menopause, circulating ovarian hormones help keep genital organs, glands, and tissues, as well as mood, primed for sexual activity. After menopause, hormone depletion coupled with aging leads to genital atrophy, which can impede sexual activity. Yet the changes linked to sexual functioning happen more slowly in some women, faster in others. Some women continue to enjoy intercourse late into life. Those who experience a debilitating decline in the sexual ability to have intercourse are happy to discover that pleasure can be gained through any number of other ways of interrelating with one's partner physically and emotionally. "You're never too old for it" is a truism—especially if partners are attuned to the enjoyment obtained from simply touching, holding, or hugging a mate as well as other sensual pleasures.

> "I get terrible hot flashes when I'm having an orgasm. It seems like the final insult. Here I'm losing the wonderful ability to have more children because of menopause, and what pleasure is left is taken away by hot flashes!"

Given the reality that sexual functioning meets up with obstacles the older a person gets, one of the best ways to ensure that physical limitations don't come between you and your partner is to communicate openly and to be emotionally reassuring.

Sexual Functioning

As seen in the last chapter, menopause-related genital changes can affect a woman's sexual ability and responsiveness. Many women wonder to what extent these changes will interfere with sexual activity as they grow older. The bottom line is that it's difficult to say, especially because conditions vary so greatly among women. Also, the whole area of sexual functioning in postmenopausal women has been only scantily researched.

For some women, signs of vaginal degeneration can appear as early as the perimenopausal years. For the majority of others, genital changes start becoming noticeable as early as one to three months after menopause. Yet a thinning of the vaginal wall and a reduction in vaginal lubrication doesn't necessarily compromise sexual activity or pleasure. In one study of women ages 45 to 65, led by Drs. Myra S. Hunter and Malcolm I. Whitehead at King's College Hospital in London, 45 percent of the postmenopausal women studied had vaginal dryness, compared to 25 percent of the premenopausal group. Yet the high level of sexual satisfaction reported overall didn't change with menopausal status. If vaginal dryness is a problem for you, there are treatments available (see Chapters 6 and 9).

Although at age 52 a woman's sexual activity may not be compromised by urogenital atrophy, problems are likely to become apparent by age 72. According to a 1990 review in the journal *Contemporary OB/GYN,* as many as 30 percent of postmenopausal women complain of painful intercourse. Other reports state that the prevalence of atrophic vaginitis (which can account for vaginal dryness, irritation, and painful intercourse) affects up to 38 percent of postmenopausal women. Postmenopausal sexual activity may be limited by a constricted vaginal opening, the clitoris's delayed response to stimulus, decreased blood flow which can further limit sexual response, fewer uterine contractions, prolapse of the vagina or uterus, and in some cases a lack of orgasm. While vaginal tissue's decline becomes more noticeable with age, a woman's general health can very much determine how severe her associated symptoms become.

Sexual Responsiveness

It's generally believed that a woman's circulating androgen affects her libido, or sexual drive, and state of arousal. The partial decline of androgen after menopause might therefore mean a partial decline in sexual responsiveness in some women. Yet there is still no direct proof that androgen influences libido. During perimenopause, even though ovarian hormone levels begin to drift lower, libido nonetheless seems intact in most women. In a prospective study of Danish women, by age 51, 70 percent of those studied reported no reduction in sexual desire. For those who did, it appeared more related to personal circumstances other than menopause.

After menopause, a woman may still retain well over 50 percent of premenopausal androgen amounts, which some researchers believe is sufficient in many women to sustain libido.

Sometimes a woman may become concerned over her lack of sexual responsiveness and worry that she has lost the ability, or even the emotion, for sex. In fact, hot flashes, vaginal dryness, or another physiological changes may be to blame. "A decline in sexual desire should not be misinterpreted as loss of sexual desire," notes Dr. Gloria

A. Bachmann, division head of Obstetrics and Gynecology at the Robert Wood Johnson University Hospital, in the 1990 *Annals of the New York Academy of Sciences.* As many women can attest, once hot flashes are alleviated through estrogen therapy, sexual desire returns.

Not infrequently, factors other than menopausal changes and more closely associated with aging may contribute to sexual dysfunction and a waning of libido. Bachmann reports that "Chronic health problems, such as cancer, arthritis, or coronary artery disease, decreased physical fitness, prior surgical procedures, unsatisfactory premenopausal sexual function, unavailability of partner, or partner sexual dysfunction" can detract from sexual activity.

Postmenopausal women need to remember that their partners are also aging and so becoming all the more susceptible to changes that affect sexual relations. For men, impotence—the inability to achieve or maintain an erection—is a common problem, one primarily associated with age-related cardiovascular deficiencies and not declining testosterone levels, as might be imagined. Sexual dysfunctioning, then, can be an early warning sign of a partner's health problem. For the sake of differentiating between medical and emotional barriers to sex, sexual counseling can be an important first step.

Surgical Menopause and Sexual Functioning

A decline in libido seems to be most noticeable in women who have undergone surgical menopause. This is probably because of the sudden reduction in androgen that the removal of the ovaries causes. Replacement androgens prescribed for such women can boost sexual desire, thoughts, and fantasies, researchers have observed.

In the short term, surgery itself takes a while to recover from, emotionally as well as physically, and can also serve to limit sexual activity. You should also be aware that if you have your uterus and/or cervix removed, this too may affect your sexual responsiveness since these organs can contribute to sexual stimulation. Over time, surgical menopause and the loss of ovarian estrogen can contribute to earlier-than-normal and more acute vaginal atrophy than if menopause had arrived naturally. The result can be reduced sexual functioning at an earlier age.

Weight Gain

Starting in midlife or shortly thereafter, a majority of women appear to gain weight, a phenomenon that many investigators believe adds to the risk for heart disease in postmenopausal women. One prospective study of 115,886 women showed that as the participants' *body mass index* (an individual's weight divided by her height) increased, there was an equivalent increase in the risk for coronary heart disease.

A survey of nearly 500 postmenopausal women codirected by Judith J. Wurtman, a research scientist at MIT, demonstrated just how extensive weight gain around the time of menopause can be. The researchers reported that 64 percent of the nonobese participants gained an average of 10 to 15 pounds after menopause. Of those who were obese before menopause, 96 percent gained an average of 21 to 23 pounds postmenopausally. Other researchers have found similar signs of postmenopausal weight gain.

Menopause and older age appear to be associated not only with increased body mass but also with a shift in fat distribution. Premenopausal women are often described as "pear-shaped," since their fat collects predominantly around their hips, thighs, and buttocks. But it's been observed that after menopause, fat deposits build up around the abdomen and tummy, lending to the "apple" shape characteristic of older men. "Apples" seem to have a higher incidence of heart disease than "pears."

Apparently, postmenopausal weight gain and weight shift are inevitable for many women. But which of the following account for these changes?

1. consuming too much high-fat food and general overeating
2. a slowdown of metabolism due to aging
3. less physical activity
4. some sort of menopause-induced alteration that influences weight change

Researchers have found reason to suspect #1, #2, and #3. And now studies are also accumulating that suggest that menopause—#4—may have a direct bearing on a decrease of lean body mass and an increase of body fat. The main evidence for this arises from a small number of studies in which hormone replacement therapy seemed to reverse weight gain in the postmenopausal years and even help maintain the lower-body pattern of fat distribution seen in younger women. If hormone supplements somehow help slow postmenopausal weight gain, menopause's hormone depletion must be playing a role in weight gain, the thinking goes. But it could also be true that women who choose to go on HRT gain less weight because they

"Before menopause I never had a weight problem, high blood pressure, or high cholesterol. Yet in the four or so years since menopause, my weight, blood pressure, and cholesterol all have progressively gone up," relates a nonetheless healthy 55-year-old woman. "I don't get it. I'm eating better than I used to—avoiding fat—and I always exercise."

take better care of themselves and would keep the pounds off even if they weren't on HRT.

What's generally agreed on is that, contrary to rumor, hormone replacement doesn't *cause* weight gain.

Since this research is in its infancy, researchers have a long way to go before they can draw conclusions. The mechanisms behind menopause-induced weight gain remain unknown. During a televised, PBS-presented discussion on menopause, Dr. Judith Reichman offered her own personal hunch: Postmenopausal weight gain, she suggested, might be nature's way of protecting a women's thinning bones.

Should research further validate menopause's direct effect on weight gain, then "menopause should be perceived as a time in women's lives when they need to be very careful about weight gain," says Wurtman of MIT. "Intervening in the perimenopausal years might be very important, especially for heavier women. Before menopause arrives, a woman might want to put special emphasis on developing and maintaining lean body mass as insurance against its later loss."

Part Two

Hormone Replacement Therapy

5

Hormone Replacement: Is It for You?

Along with many other women, you're probably concerned about whether to take estrogen, progestin, or androgen supplements. Are they safe? Do women actually need them? After all, haven't we survived millennia just fine without them? Are doctors "medicalizing" a natural part of life that's no big deal? The answers to these questions will differ from individual to individual, but they all deserve a closer look.

First, a brief definition may be helpful: Hormone replacement therapy, or HRT, generally refers to so-called exogenous sex hormones—that is, estrogens, progestins, or androgens that are medically introduced into the body to replace the ovarian-made hormones depleted by menopause.

Is HRT the right choice for you? If so, what combination of hormones is best for you? When should you avoid HRT? If you decide to try this therapy, when should you

"I'm on hormones because tests showed I've undergone some bone loss. But I'm not wholeheartedly in agreement with taking hormones. It feels very experimental, like we don't really know all the answers."

begin it, and for how long should you stay on it? This and the following chapter will give you the information you need to make an informed decision. We'll start with a brief overview before focusing on individual choices.

Do you need supplemental hormones for perimenopause? Since the ovaries' hormonal output begins receding years before menopause, some women may benefit from replacement hormones before menopause to relieve menopausal symptoms, particularly hot flashes and irregular bleeding.

For many physicians, the low-dose birth control pill represents the treatment of choice for women whose perimenopausal symptoms are severe. The Pill contains greater amounts of estrogens and progestins than those found in HRT doses commonly prescribed after menopause. Because of this higher dosage, the Pill works to block the pituitary gland's stimulation of ovarian hormone production. Hence, it turns off the natural menstrual cycle while producing an artificial menstrual cycle and becoming the body's main source of estrogens and progestins. By putting a full quota of hormones back into the system, the Pill relieves hot flashes and other menopausal symptoms caused by estrogen depletion. Used prior to menopause, it can also serve as a handy provider of contraception during a time in life when women are surprised to learn that they can still easily become pregnant. If a woman smokes, the Pill will be ruled out because of the associated increased risk of stroke and heart attack. Also, it should be noted that users of the Pill run the risk of phlebitis, the inflammation of a vein, which places a person at risk for a blood clot.

If you choose replacement hormones after menopause, you'll find that standard postmenopausal HRT doses are lower than those contained in low-dose birth control pills. Some women wonder whether they should go on these lower HRT doses before menopause in order to counter-act perimenopause's decreasing levels of hormones. If your symptoms aren't all that disruptive and you still have menstrual bleeding, doctors generally believe that you don't need perimenopausal HRT. The very activity of menstrual bleeding signifies that your body is still produc-ing an adequate level of hormones. Also, such low hor-mone doses taken premenopausally can be problematic. Unlike the Pill, they don't block the body's natural men-strual cycling. Therefore, you would be getting a double dose of hormones—those made by your ovaries plus those provided through medication. Your bleeding, then, would result from two different hormonal sources.

One form of HRT is estrogen replacement therapy, or ERT. This refers to the administration of supplemental es-trogens only. As will be further described in Chapter 7, most postmenopausal women who take hormone replace-ment don't take estrogens alone. Instead, they take an HRT combination—usually estrogens and progestins, or estrogens, progestins, and androgens. The inclusion of progestins dates back to the late 1970s after reports began surfacing that women with an intact uterus who were tak-ing estrogens alone showed a higher incidence of endome-trial cancer. Progestins in the presence of estrogens, researchers now know, offset this increased risk. ERT, then, is largely reserved for women who have had their uterus removed.

An Individualized Approach to HRT

Some health professionals are reluctant to recommend hormone replacement therapy. If older women needed them for some reason, nature would have provided women with a full quota of sex hormones until the day they die. There's also the worry that not enough is known about estrogen's connection to cancer and HRT's long-term risks.

On the other hand, many other practitioners—including this author—feel that at this stage in its research history, hormone replacement therapy appears to represent a relatively safe and effective medical aid. It should be noted that HRT-associated medical problems that arose in the past often proved to be related to *dose* and not content. Today HRT seems to be especially appropriate for post-menopausal women who are at a higher risk for osteoporosis and possibly for those at a higher risk for heart disease. Because women, on average, are living for many more postmenopausal years than previously, they are all the more susceptible to conditions linked to prolonged lower levels of estrogen. There is, in fact, wide agreement that the medical community needs many more large, randomized, controlled studies for greater insight into HRT's longer-term influence on cells and systems. Several major studies are already under way for that very reason. Nonetheless, the research so far conducted includes thousands of reports submitted worldwide. These indicate that ERT and HRT generally appear to pose more benefits than risks for appropriate candidates.

If you're considering HRT for whatever reasons, I need to emphasize and reemphasize that the decision is a personal one. It should be based on your individualized health needs as well as your own assessment of HRT's benefits. A doctor's role is to present you with information, and this book should be of assistance. But the responsibility of making the best choice possible ultimately rests with you. Since in most cases HRT is considered elective, you should be aware of its risks as well as its benefits.

While hormone replacement can present many women with a valuable opportunity for enhancing their health in later years, HRT is not for everyone. Your body simply may not need supplemental hormones. Or because of past or present health conditions, you may not be able to use them. A wise diet, regular exercise, vacation time, a little TLC, and other health maintainers may be all your body requires.

Do You Really Need HRT?

Are you healthy and active? Are you sailing through the symptoms of menopause? Are you fortunate enough to have no increased risk for osteoporosis or heart disease as indicated by your family history and your personal health history? If you can answer "yes" to these three questions, then there's no compelling reason to take replacement hormones.

Active women of medium to heavy build who don't smoke usually maintain a better defense against osteoporosis in their later years than thinner women. Hence they may have less need for hormone therapy. Overweight women, in particular, may not require hormones, since they're likely to produce higher levels of postmenopausal estrogens than slimmer women. In addition, the estrogen circulating in postmenopausal overweight women is apt to be more potent. Because these women appear to have less of a certain protein that binds to estrogen in the bloodstream, the estrogen in their systems tends to be more active.

Aside from any of the above considerations, you may decide against HRT because you feel unsure of or are strongly opposed to hormone therapy or drug use in general. A majority of women still let perimenopause, menopause, and postmenopause run their natural courses without hormone intervention. Others opt for alternative treatments to help alleviate specific troubling symptoms, such as hot flashes, or to treat longer-term concerns, including bone loss. (See Part Three for suggestions.)

When HRT May Not Be the Choice for You

Supplemental hormones, particularly estrogens, can heighten the risk of certain known or suspected medical conditions and therefore are not recommended in certain cases. If you're contemplating HRT but have a condition that may indicate against its use, the risks will need to be closely weighed by you and your family doctor and gynecologist, as well as by any specialists (for example, an oncologist or cardiologist) from whom you've received care.

Conditions that may rule out the use of replacement hormones include suspected endometrial or breast cancer, a history of vaginal cancer, active liver disease, undiagnosed genital bleeding, or an indication of blood-clotting (thromboembolic) disease. (See Chapter 6 for a full review of these disease-related risks.)

Not long ago, past episodes of endometrial cancer, breast cancer, and blood clotting were usually considered reasons to advise against hormone therapy. But little by little, doctors are prescribing HRT in such cases, with no negative side effects reported. In women with a past history of endometrial cancer, estrogen therapy appears to be tolerated with no evidence of increased recurrence. For some women with a history of blood clotting, there's evidence that HRT, because it is low-dose, doesn't increase the risk of blood clots the way the birth control pill does. (In such cases, doctors usually recommend nonoral routes for estrogens, such as the skin patch, instead of swallowed tablets. Nonoral routes avoid the liver wherein blood-clotting factors arise.) Finally, when estrogens are prescribed for breast cancer survivors, no strong data shows that appropriate doses cause a reactivation of the disease. There is even some indication that women with breast cancer who took ERT before they were diagnosed do better in the long run than those who were never on estrogens.

Depending on the severity and history of the disorder, several other conditions may dictate against HRT or cause a doctor to question its use. These include gallbladder disease, high blood pressure (hypertension), the presence of fibroids or endometriosis, diabetes, and acute porphyria, which is a metabolic disorder.

Smoking is not a contraindication for estrogen doses commonly used after menopause. However, if you smoke, you should not take birth control pills—neither for contraceptive purposes nor for perimenopausal symptoms. Their significantly higher doses of hormones lead to an increased potential for blood clotting that can be amplified by smoking's tendency to constrict blood vessels. Since smoking is associated with increased risk of heart disease and cancer, among other diseases, you should quit as soon as possible. Ask your doctor about support and recommendations for a good program for quitting.

Could You Clearly Benefit from HRT?

If you're at a higher-than-average risk for osteoporosis or manifest any components of heart disease—particularly atherosclerosis—or you are troubled by persistent hot flashes and symptoms that signal acute vaginal atrophy, these may be significant reasons for considering therapeu-

> "I have a family history of heart disease. Even though replacement estrogens might add extra protection against heart disease, I haven't wanted to use them because the birth control pill's estrogen used to give me migraines. Recently I had a thallium test [which tests for heart function]. It turned up no signs of heart problems, so I really don't feel as though I need estrogens."

tic hormones. Physicians also often recommend HRT and ERT for women who have undergone an early natural menopause or who have had their ovaries surgically removed. Because these women face more years of lower ovarian hormone levels than those undergoing menopause later in life, they are all the more vulnerable to conditions linked to hormone deficiency.

Making the Decision

For some of you, the decision of whether or not to begin hormone replacement can be clear-cut. If you have two sisters who have been diagnosed with breast cancer, which some investigators believe to be an estrogen-related can-cer, you will probably be opposed to hormone use. There is a chance that you share a genetic susceptibility to that cancer, which theoretically might be triggered by pro-longed exposure to estrogens. On the other hand, if you experienced premature menopause at age 37 and your mother was diagnosed with spinal osteoporosis, you may unhesitatingly choose HRT.

> "In the early 1980s, six months after beginning estrogen therapy, my sister was found to have breast cancer. For that reason, when I reached menopause, I decided never to take estrogens, and I've never wavered."

For most women, the factors weighed in reaching this decision won't be as dramatically clear-cut. You may want to begin replacement therapy for cosmetic reasons, per-suaded by reports that estrogen can slow the skin's wrin-kling and thinning and preserve a pear-shaped figure. Bear in mind, however, that hormones can't be recommended for cosmetic reasons alone. You and your health-care provider should analyze your family's health history, your individual health background and status, and your health-related habits: Do you exercise? Do you eat the right foods? A total health review will provide a forecast of your future health and indicate whether or not hormone therapy will serve a health-related purpose. If you're still undecided, the following considerations might help.

To be most effective, an HRT program must be followed strictly.

This might seem a minor consideration compared to whether or not you need to go on HRT in the first place. However, like many people who take prescribed medications, many women who elect to go on HRT don't keep up with their drug-taking schedules. So it pays to look at all the reasons. Going on HRT for less than a year may quell hot flashes and temporarily assuage vaginal atrophy. But to achieve HRT's full benefits—treatment for longer-lasting symptoms and protection against heart disease and osteoporosis—generally requires a commitment of several years. Ongoing studies of women on HRT—for example, HERS (the Heart & Estrogen-Progestin Replacement Study) and the NIH's Women's Health Initiative—should add insight into what length treatment offers maximum benefits.

An analysis of the Medication Use Studies Data Base conducted by the University of Mississippi discovered how widespread HRT noncompliance is. It found that 57 percent of women on estrogen replacement "fail to take their medication properly." According to a separate report, 20 percent of new HRT users stop taking their prescribed medication within nine months and from 20 to 30 percent never have their prescriptions filled. Of the many reasons for noncompliance, women often cite the inconvenience of returning to monthly bleeding. (As Chapter 7 describes, this side effect accompanies one HRT administration regimen.) HRT also can bring back the periodic mood swings, breast tenderness, and bloating that a woman thought she had left behind with her last natural period. Breakthrough bleeding can be yet another undesirable side effect. Although changes in how HRT is used can help many users move beyond HRT's unwanted effects, many women's patience understandably wears thin before they arrive at a more accommodating HRT approach.

> "When I first went on hormones, the schedule called for 10 mg of Provera [a progestin] the latter part of each month. Right after starting, I turned into a jumping bean—totally hyper. Also, I was constantly upset or grouchy—filled with all these terrible demons. And I couldn't sleep. I was just a mess. After two weeks of going crazy, I called my doctor and he lowered the dose to 5 mg and thankfully that returned me to normal."

Frequently, a woman's fear of an HRT-associated increased risk of breast cancer may discourage her from continuing hormone therapy. Discussing risk factors with your doctor and reviewing the significant findings published in the medical literature can help you decide. (See Chapter 6 for a discussion of HRT and the risk of breast cancer.) It's best not to begin HRT unless you fully trust its outcome; if you're skeptical or uncertain, you're less likely to follow the treatment schedule.

Finally, taking any medication on a regular basis can be a chore. Consequently, you may frequently forget to take it or stop taking it altogether. "When I was put on antibiotics, I found I couldn't keep up with the pill-taking schedule—and I'm a nurse!" points out Mary A. Riordan, a registered nurse within the MGH's Department of Gynecology. When HRT is administered orally, in tablet form, women often have two different bottles of pills (estrogens and progestins) to think about, and sometimes two different medication schedules. "It can be confusing and seemingly time-consuming, especially for women who aren't used to taking pills," says Riordan. If you opt for supplemental hormones, you should be prepared to adhere to a consistent medication routine. Newly approved products that package oral estrogens and progestins together for pill-taking convenience may help women keep on schedule. (See Chapter 7.)

For those of you who aren't good pill takers, the *transdermal* (through the skin) administration of estrogens via a skin patch may simplify life. It's guesstimated that estrogen patches, which are changed once or twice a week, are associated with a higher rate of compliance than oral estrogens. Transdermal progestins aren't yet approved in the United States. So if you want to avoid progestins in pill form, you can opt for progestins that can be injected intramuscularly or used vaginally in suppository form. (See Chapter 7.)

Look into Alternatives

If you have no clear-cut health reason to choose hormone replacement, yet you want protection over time from many postmenopausal body changes, nonhormonal therapy may be the way to go. Even when there are reasons for going with HRT, a woman may find that her questions and qualms about HRT predispose her toward an alternative approach. For those whose medical conditions cancel out HRT, nonhormonal treatment can be the only choice. (See Section Three.)

Within this category you'll find drugs well tested by Western medicine. You'll also find alternative measures, such as Western or Chinese herbal approaches that currently lack firm scientific validation yet are supported by anecdotal reports. Long overdue, more attention is being paid to alternative medicine, as reflected by new research outlets such as the NIH's Center for Alternative Medicine and the Richard and Hinda Rosenthal Center for Alternative/Complementary Medicine at Columbia University. As a result, we can all look forward to a better appraisal of alternative approaches in the years ahead.

A Bone Density Test Can Help You Decide

If you're contemplating HRT, having your bone's mineral content and bone strength tested can aid you in your decision. A bone densitometry test serves as a helpful indicator of a woman's susceptibility to osteoporosis. If your bone density is below what's considered healthy for your age, it can be a sign of *osteopenia,* or bone loss. Estrogen supplements or other treatment may be called for in order to curb bone loss, particularly the rapid loss that occurs in the first few years after menopause.

If your bone density is equal to or above the norm, you may not need hormone replacement—at least not for the time being and not for bone loss. A normal reading at the time of menopause, however, does not guarantee that you'll be osteoporosis-free in the future. If HRT hasn't been prescribed, it's useful to undergo the same testing one to two years later in order to check the rate of bone loss. You should consider additional bone testing every two to three years thereafter.

Several different methods test for bone density, with newer techniques being easier to use and giving more precise, accurate, and reproducible results. (Note that a *bone density measurement* is very different from a *bone scan,* a test that evaluates the activity of bone cells and is often used for scanning for cancer.) MGH osteoporosis specialist Dr. Robert M. Neer currently recommends testing of the spine or hip by *dual-energy X-ray absorptiometry* (DEXA or DXA), a technique developed in the late 1980s. DXA is more sensitive to early bone loss than older methods and offers shorter scan times (a few minutes, at most), clearer images and less radiation exposure. It allows for the evaluation of two important types of bone—cortical and trabecular. During the postmenopausal years, signs of osteoporosis are detected first in *trabecular* bone, the porous inner bone found in spinal vertebrae, the top of the hip and the ends of leg and arm bones. *Cortical* bone, which often sheathes trabecular bone, is also vulnerable to osteopenia, especially bone loss that arises from certain endocrine disorders such as overactive parathyroid glands. With more limited techniques such as single photon absorptiometry, only cortical bone is measured.

Approved by the FDA in 1993, *quantitative computed tomography* (QCT) represents the most precise diagnostic method. Trained on the forearm bone, a QCT machine (in essence, a miniature CT scanner that produces three-dimensional images) can detect very early signs of osteoporosis not always visible with older technology. Unlike other devices, QCT can zero in on trabecular bone and measure it separately and distinctly from cortical bone.

QCT, however, is quite expensive, which can limit its use for patient care. Approximate costs for QCT vary from $150 to $300. DXA can be slightly less expensive ($150 to $200). But costs for bone measurement, no matter the technique used, vary greatly from state to state, as does available coverage from health insurance providers.

Conventional lumbar and thoracic X rays are useful in detecting spine abnormalities such as fracture. They can also spot bone loss. However, osteoporotic changes don't normally show up on conventional X rays until as much as 30 percent of skeletal calcium has been lost. As for the once-common bone-testing technique known as dual-photon absorptiometry, it has been surpassed by newer methods.

All the newer methods in use take under fifteen minutes to perform. None cause pain or discomfort.

Looking ahead, other bone densitometry techniques are being developed, including ultrasound, the technology that uses high-frequency sound waves to produce images of internal structures. For now, however, ultrasound's adaptation to bone imaging is still being worked out. Ultrasound, unlike the other methods described, would use no radiation. Routine bone densitometer measurements by DXA or single-photon absorptiometry utilize radiation exposures that are as low-level as the high-altitude radiation a person receives when flying across the country. QCTs on the forearm produce slightly higher radiation levels. Conventional X rays and QCTs used on the spine, however, use even higher levels of radiation.

Ideally, if you choose to take a bone density test, your physician should recommend a method based on its scan reproducability, accuracy, precision, and radiation dose, as well as the bone (e.g., spine, hip, or forearm) being measured.

Current Studies

Despite the years of validating research on hormone replacement therapy, it will never be completely free of uncertainties until further long-term investigation is complete. Someday, based on more thorough research, the choice of whether or not to employ HRT should be much more clear-cut.

Among several ongoing studies, the NIH's Women's Health Initiative represents a significant move in this direction. Unfortunately, its data won't be available until after the year 2005. Enrolling approximately 63,000 women between the ages of 50 and 79, the initiative's primary intent is to study the effects of hormone therapy on heart disease, breast cancer, and osteoporosis. Also being evaluated is the impact of supplemental calcium and vitamin D and a low-fat diet on postmenopausal health. One stumbling block this study may face is noncompliance. Some sources contend that the high rate of women who initiate, then drop, hormone therapy could hamper the initiative's outcome.

Clinical trial data from the Heart & Estrogen-Progestin Replacement Study (HERS) will reach us sooner, but will shed light only on the shorter-term effects of HRT on heart disease. Recruiting 2,340 postmenopausal women with coronary heart disease (CHD), HERS researchers are testing the supposition that HRT can reduce the risk of death in women with CHD by as much as 80 percent. Coordinated by researchers at the University of California/San Francisco, the study will be in progress for nearly five years.

The results of the three-year Postmenopausal Estrogen/Progestin Interventions (PEPI) trial, announced in late 1994, have added support to the finding that estrogens taken alone or combined with progestins can carry substantial lipid benefits which may infer cardiovascular benefits. While PEPI, sponsored by five NIH institutes, seems to confirm HRT's positive impact on blood cholesterol, the study's brief duration precluded it from drawing any conclusion about HRT's long-term influence on cardiovascular health.

Since its 1948 beginnings, the Framingham Heart Study (headquartered in Framingham, Massachusetts) has been probing the risk factors for vascular disease through an initial cohort of 5,209 men and women, with a second cohort of 5,135 offspring of the original study subjects more recently added. With cardiac health in mind, Framingham researchers have looked at women's natural history of menopause, with some studies assessing hormone replacement therapy's effects on heart and bone. Supported by NIH funding through 2001, future Framingham observations undoubtedly will contribute to a broader understanding of postmenopausal changes, as will two other long-running surveys—the Nurses' Health Study and the Massachusetts Women's Health Study.

Also backed by NIH dollars, the Nurses' study has been following health changes in thousands of female registered nurses since 1976. The study started with approximately 122,000 participants, age 30 to 55, and subsequently has added new participants. Many of the nurses have since traversed menopause. Consequently, the survey has proved a major source for reports on postmenopausal changes and changes associated with hormone replacement.

Begun in 1981, the Massachusetts Women's Health Study was primarily designed to study the natural menopause transition and continues to generate information on the physiological changes associated with menopause, as well as the effects of HRT. Its study participants include a random sample of over 400 Massachusetts women, many of whom were initially premenopausal but have since undergone menopause. The study is funded by the NIH's National Institute on Aging and is being di-

Table 1. Techniques for Measuring Bone Density

TECHNIQUE (ALPHABETICALLY)	BONES MEASURED	EXAM TIME (MINUTES)	POSSIBLE ACCURACY ERROR (%)	EFFECTIVE RADIATION DOSE (μ SV)*
Dual Energy X-ray Absorptiometry (DXA) uses a double beam from an X-ray source	Spine Hip, Total Body	10–20	3–9	1
Dual Photon Absorptiometry DPA uses a double beam from a radioactive energy source	Spine, Hip, Total Body	20–40	4–10	5
Quantitative Computed Tomography (QCT) uses a conventional CT scanner with specialized software	Spine	10–15	5–20	60**
Peripheral QCT (pQCT) is a special version of the QCT that measures only the bone density of the wrist	Wrist	10	4–8	3
Radiographic Absorptiometry (RA) uses an X ray of the hand and a small metal wedge to calculate bone density	Hand	1–3	4	1
Single Energy X-ray Absorptiometry (SXA) uses an X-ray source to measure bone	Wrist, Heel	4	5	<1
Single Photon Absorptiometry (SPA) uses a single beam from an energy source passed through water	Wrist	15	4–6	<1

* Effective dose refers to radiation that reaches internal organs. For comparison, one chest X ray gives a radiation dose of about 50 μSv, a lateral-spin X ray 500 to 1,000 μSv, an abdominal CT scan about 4,000 μSv, and natural background radiation is about 2,000 to 3,000 μSv per year.

** Radiation dose may be up to 600 μSv on older CT scanners.

Table: National Osteoporosis Foundation.

rected by researchers at the New England Research Institutes in Watertown, Massachusetts.

While the definitive total picture of hormone replacement therapy is still many years off, there is an ever-growing body of information and resources to help you make as informed a decision as possible. Seek out details about the associated benefits and risks, as well as alternative therapies, from physicians and the medical literature. Chapter 11's "Resources" suggests journals, newsletters, books, videos, institutions, and other sources that can provide helpful input.

Many women wonder if they can trust the drug companies and their PR materials—pamphlets, books, videos, and spot advertisements—to provide reliable, unbiased information on HRT products. Generally, the specifics these companies provide are scientifically accurate, since advertised materials are monitored by the FDA. Yet it's also self-evident that drug companies are trying to sell their products, and you shouldn't let the promoted features in a magazine ad outweigh a clear understanding of a product's associated risks. Then again, due to stringent FDA regulations, those risks are so strongly spelled out in the directions that accompany an HRT product that doctors sometimes complain it scares off patients from following through with the taking of a needed prescription.

For more information on weighing the pros and cons of HRT, please see the next chapter.

6

Weighing the Benefits and Risks of Hormone Replacement Therapy

As science advances, uncertainty nearly always dogs its steps. With dramatic breakthroughs come errors, most often manifested in long-term developments impossible to foresee. One high-profile reminder of medicine's fallibility is DES (diethylstilbestrol), the estrogenlike synthetic compound pregnant women took in the 1940s and 1950s to prevent miscarriages. By 1971 DES had become implicated in a higher than usual rate of a rare vaginal cancer in the daughters of DES-treated women. Banned that year for use in pregnancy maintenance, today a better understood DES is a treatment option for prostate cancer, although more effective medications are usually used.

There have been other tragic, unpredictable outcomes. The high incidence of heart attacks in the 1970s among younger women on the Pill who smoked was later linked to the early Pill's high estrogen content. Also in that same decade came a rise of endometrial cancer among women on estrogen therapy. Later it became clear that, in order to maintain a premenopausal women's natural hormone balance, supplemental progestins were needed to offset the increased risk of uterine cancer posed by estrogen given alone.

Despite past mistakes, medicine continuously makes progress. Even the drugs with which it has erred have had their benefits. Nonetheless, any drug that has posed problems in the past—such as estrogen—is likely to raise skepticism. Is hormone therapy some kind of grand experiment? Could it be that ten or twenty years down the road, some unforeseen health calamity will arise due to the hormonal compounds we're processing in the laboratory?

The good news about HRT today is that its benefits appear to outweigh its risks. And the risks seem sufficiently understood so that many physicians, including this author, feel it's medically sound, even advisable, to prescribe hormones when a patient will benefit from their use. Over thirty years' research stands behind supplemental estrogens, which says something about medicine's understanding and belief in hormone replacement. Still, although many in the medical community hold a positive view of HRT, only continued research can provide the definite proof, the final word.

One aspect of HRT that women question most is its effects on breast cancer. As will be reviewed later in this chapter, current research gives no clear sense that the use of appropriate doses of estrogens has added significantly to the number of breast cancer cases diagnosed in this country. However, some studies have shown small increases in incidence among some longer-term users. A second concern is that progestins, when taken in combination with estrogens, can reduce the protection against heart disease estrogens provide. Although this may be true of some types of progestins, their effect doesn't seem to totally negate the positive cardiac influence of estrogens. No matter the progestin used, the outcome of estrogen-progestin combinations appears to help protect against heart disease and improve users' quality of life. One type of progestin—micronized progesterone—may provide the most noticeable benefit for cholesterol, according to the recently concluded PEPI trial.

Estrogens' poor track record in the past largely sprang from birth control pill and replacement therapy doses that were excessively high, coupled with a lack of scientific data on the cancer risks of unopposed estrogens (that is, estrogens taken alone) for women with a uterus. We now know that smaller amounts of exogenous estrogens can achieve the same benefits previously gained through larger doses, and current practice reflects this knowledge. Between 1974 and 1981, prescribed daily doses of estrogens dropped significantly, as reported by one survey of physicians. Doses fell from an average of 1.25 mg (milligrams) in 1974 to 0.625 mg in 1981. In the late 1960s and early 1970s, it wasn't uncommon for physicians to prescribe daily oral estrogen doses three to four times higher than what's commonly prescribed today.

By further comparison, the standard oral dosage currently used for postmenopausal hormone therapy—0.625 mg conjugated equine estrogens (CEE) at the level of the liver—is equivalent in potency to one-quarter of the ethinyl estradiol used in today's birth control pill. Moreover, today's Pill contains roughly one-third of the estrogen found in the Pill of the 1960s.

How does the commonly used oral dose of 0.625 mg

Figure 7. Oral Contraceptive Estrogen Content

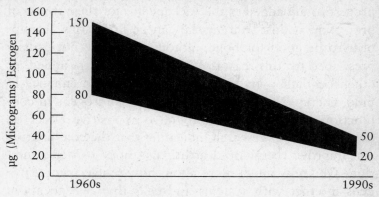

The estrogen content in oral contraceptives has been reduced over the past three decades. Dose-response studies show that lower dosages of estrogen are equally effective as the older, higher dosages.

Source: *Menopause Management*, November/December 1992.

CEE compare to what's circulating in a woman's system before menopause? On balance, it's considered to be the same as or less than the premenopausal ovaries' daily output of estrogen. This dose is thought to be the minimal effective dose to achieve bone and cardiovascular protection. However, lower doses may be adequate for relief of hot flashes and vaginal dryness.

The Basic Hormone Replacement Regimen

For most women on HRT, replacement estrogens represent the core medication in their replacement package, because of their demonstrated ability to maintain heart and bone health and reduce menopausal symptoms. When progestins are added to the package, it's for the purpose of protecting against endometrial cancer. Progestins also appear to be good for bone, although they are not usually prescribed for this reason. When androgens are added, or taken on their own, their purpose is to help enhance libido, energy, or a sense of well-being. Androgens in conjunction with estrogens also have a positive effect on bone, with some research indicating that the combination can improve rheumatoid arthritis, a bone-related condition. We know much more about how replacement estrogens interact with systems and cells than we do about replacement progestins and androgens. However, current dosages of these two hormones are generally deemed safe in appropriate circumstances.

Estrogens, although FDA-approved for the treatment of menopausal hot flashes, vaginal dryness, and bone loss, have not received FDA approval for the treatment of heart disease. Yet, just as many other drugs are used for nonapproved indications, physicians regularly prescribe estrogens in cases where the hormone can benefit a woman's cardiac health. Similarly, while progestins are approved as treatment for irregular uterine bleeding, they aren't approved for protection against endometrial cancer. Still, based on research findings, physicians routinely couple them with estrogens for this purpose. Androgens are federally approved for the treatment of a low sex drive in men but lack the same approval for treatment in women due to the need for more research.

The following table of generics represents the most commonly taken estrogens, progestins, and androgens.

Table 2. Commonly Prescribed Estrogens, Progestins, and Androgens

	Manufacturer	Product Name
Oral (by Mouth) Estrogens		
micronized estradiol	Mead Johnson	Estrace
esterified estrogen	Solvay	Estratab
conjugated equine estrogens	Wyeth-Ayerst	Premarin
estropipate	Upjohn	Ogen
	Ortho	Ortho-Est
ethinyl estradiol	Schering	Estinyl
quinestrol	Parke-Davis	Estrovis
Transdermal (through the skin) Estrogens		
transdermal estradiol	Ciba	Estraderm
	Berlex/3M	Climara
Estrogen Vaginal Creams		
17 beta-estradiol	Mead Johnson	Estrace Vaginal Cream
estropipate	Upjohn	Ogen Vaginal Cream
conjugated equine estrogens	Wyeth-Ayerst	Premarin Vaginal Cream
dienestrol	Ortho	Ortho Dienestrol Cream
dienestrol	Solvay	Estragard Cream
Estrogen Injections		
estradiol cypionate	Upjohn	Depo-Estradiol
estradiol valerate	Mead Johnson	Delestrogen
estradiol valerate	Solvay	Estraval
Oral Progestins		
medroxyprogesterone acetate	Upjohn	Provera
	Solvay	Curretab
	Wyeth-Ayerst	Cycrin
	Carnrick	Amen
norethindrone acetate	Wyeth-Ayerst	Aygestin
	Parke-Davis	Norlutate
norethindrone	Ortho	Micronor
	Syntex	Nor-Q.D.
	Parke-Davis	Norlutin
norgestrel	Wyeth-Ayerst	Ovrette

Table 2 (continued)

	MANUFACTURER	PRODUCT NAME
megesterol acetate	Bristol-Myers Squibb	Megace
progesterone micronized powder	(produced by various labs)	
Vaginal Progestins		
progesterone vaginal suppositories		
Progestin Injections		
progesterone in oil	(produced by various labs)	
Oral Androgens		
methyltestosterone	ICN	Android-10
fluoxymesterone	Upjohn	Halotestin
	Solvay	Fluoxymesterone
Androgen Injections		
testosterone enanthate	Gynex	Delatestryl
testosterone cypionate	Upjohn	Depo-Testosterone
Oral Estrogen-Androgen Combinations		
conjugated equine estrogens plus methyltestosterone	Wyeth-Ayerst	Premarin with Methyltestosterone
esterified estrogens plus methyltestosterone	Solvay	Estratest

BASIC MEDICATION TIPS

• The widely used dose of 0.625 milligrams (mg)/day of oral conjugated equine estrogens, or an equivalent dose of a different type of estrogen, has been shown to effectively lower the risk of heart disease as well as to treat a range of disorders, including hot flashes, vaginal dryness, and bone loss.

• If you go on estrogens and your uterus is intact, you'll probably also need to take progestins for protection against estrogen-provoked endometrial growth. In a very small number of cases, excess growth of the uterine lining can ultimately result in cancer. It isn't yet known how low a dose of progestins serves to offset the risk to the endometrium. To be on the safe side, physicians often prescribe 10 mg/day of oral medroxyprogesterone acetate or an equivalent dose of a different progestin in tandem with estrogens. However, there's a growing trend toward using lower doses—5 mg, and even 2.5 mg—as long as the endometrial lining displays no overgrowth. In the 1970s, when the medical community became alarmed over the increased incidence of endometrial abnormalities associated with unopposed estrogens, physicians may have overreacted. Higher doses of progestins may be unnecessary and may only exacerbate unwanted side effects, such as mood swings and breast tenderness.

Hormone Therapy and Heart Disease

Had you asked your doctor in the 1950s if estrogen therapy could protect you against heart disease in your postmenopausal years, in all likelihood he or she would have given you a thumbs-up sign. Back then, estrogens were enthusiastically touted as "fountains of youth and protectors against heart disease." By the 1970s, however, your doctor would have given you an unequivocal thumbs-down. In the mid-1960s the Coronary Drug Project had found that high-dose estrogens prescribed to men resulted in more nonfatal *myocardial infarctions* (heart attacks), pulmonary emboli, and deaths than a placebo. More worrisome news came in the mid-1970s, when British investigators observed an above-normal incidence of heart attacks in young women taking high-estrogen contraceptives, and a Boston University researcher reported a fourfold risk of heart attack among female estrogen users as compared to nonusers, with estrogen implicated in both cases.

Today, however, in response to the same question most doctors would again be giving the thumbs-up sign. Once more, the pendulum has swung in favor of estrogen as a cardiac protector. Ever since estrogen doses in both contraceptives and replacement therapy began decreasing in the mid-1970s, more recent epidemiologic studies report that postmenopausal women taking estrogens do, in fact, have a lower rate of heart disease than untreated women. Some reports suggest as much as a 50 percent reduction in risk.

With the pendulum of opinion having swung so radically in the past, is the current optimism reliable? Yes, up to a point. Some caution is advised in assuming that estrogens will reduce your risk of heart disease by as much as 50 percent. The risk reduction for each individual may be less dramatic. Nevertheless, if estrogens lower your risk by only 10 percent, this would still amount to a significant impact on public health.

In explanation, let's first take a look at the findings. Estrogens' therapeutic value to the circulatory system appears strongly linked to its ability to thwart atherosclerotic disease, or the buildup of plaque on the inner walls of coronary vessels. Yet how it does this remains uncertain. Studies have shown that orally administered estrogens can elevate high-density lipoproteins (HDL), the "good" lipoproteins, by as much as 10 to 18 percent, and reduce low-density lipoproteins (LDL), the "bad" lipoproteins, by 10 to 19 percent. Recent data also suggest that estrogens may impact cardiac health in several other ways. Little is known about how estrogens directly benefit blood vessels, but they appear to impede the uptake of LDL cholesterol through artery walls, thereby lowering the chances for plaque formation associated with atherosclerosis. Plaque-restricted arteries, which impede the flow of blood-carried oxygen to the heart muscles, can result in angina (chest pain), heart attack, and other circulation disorders. By reducing plaque, estrogens appear to lessen the incidence of both heart attack and angina. There's evidence that they also enlarge artery pathways, enhance blood flow, and generally benefit the workings of both arterial and heart muscles.

One negative aspect: Exogenous estrogens may elevate triglycerides, lipids in the blood that, at high levels, can lead to heart disease. If your triglyceride levels are already high, this might warrant a more careful approach to HRT.

Since the 1980s, several studies of postmenopausal women have shown that those taking estrogens have one-third to one-half the risk of heart attack than women not on estrogens. Data derived from a ten-year follow-up of 48,470 postmenopausal women from the Nurses' Health Study also posted positive results. The 1991 report stated that women taking estrogens had a 44 percent reduction in risk for coronary disease compared to the expected risk. In contrast, the Framingham Heart Study found notably higher rates of cardiovascular and cerebrovascular disease among estrogen users compared to nonusers. After reanalysis, however, these findings were considered invalid. Overall, methodology problems have been cited in connection with the few studies that show an increased risk for heart disease among estrogen users. A 1996 study of women at the Kaiser Permanente group in California found that women who had taken estrogens had less heart disease, but the effect showed up only after fifteen years of use.

Let's revisit the statistic that estrogen therapy can reduce heart disease by as much as 50 percent. Bear in mind that this figure is mostly derived from research involving women who tend to be healthy and health conscious to begin with. Through their own initiative they enrolled in estrogen therapy and kept on it. Very possibly, then, non-estrogen-related factors made these study participants less prone to heart disease than the general population to begin with. For a truer picture of risk reduction, studies that use a random selection of women are needed.

Subcategories of Heart Disease

Of the various disorders lumped within the broad category of heart disease, estrogens appear to be particularly effective for those linked to atherosclerosis. *Ischemic heart disease,* a cardiac disorder caused by the narrowing of arteries and a related impasse of blood-bearing oxygen, often originates from atherosclerosis, as does *myocardial infarction* (heart attack). Estrogens taken by women after menopause have been associated with a reduction in ischemic heart disease and myocardial infarction, as well as lower total cholesterol and reduced atherosclerosis.

Cerebrovascular disease—which is responsible for brain-related circulatory disorders, notably stroke—can also be caused by atherosclerosis. While studies of estrogens' effects on stroke have yielded conflicting data, there is reassuring evidence that hormone therapy doesn't increase the risk for stroke and, in the future, might even be shown to be a preventive for stroke. One 1988 prospective study of 8,882 women in a California retirement community showed fewer deaths from stroke among estrogen users versus nonusers. In a separate study, Swedish researchers studied 23,088 women who had been prescribed estrogens from 1977 to 1980 and concluded that more potent strengths of estrogens appeared to reduce the risk of stroke, especially when started shortly after menopause. On the other hand, some studies have discovered no change in stroke incidence between estrogen users and nonusers.

High Blood Pressure

High blood pressure, or hypertension, can be caused or intensified by a number of different circumstances, including thyroid and kidney disorders, a high cholesterol level, and obesity. While it may not stem directly from a circulatory problem, high blood pressure can lead to stroke or heart attack, and is therefore often studied together with cardiovascular disorders.

If you have high blood pressure, your physician most likely will want your condition brought under control before prescribing estrogens, since they could possibly aggravate symptoms. However, data from the PEPI trial show that neither unopposed estrogens nor estrogens combined with progestins appears to raise blood pressure, at least within a three-year period. New insights also suggest that women who have previously experienced high blood pressure may actually benefit from hormone replacement, given evidence that estrogens may be capable of reducing the incidence of stroke and some of its causes.

Estrogen Therapy and a History of Heart Disease

Women on estrogens with a history of heart disease may have fewer heart problems and improve their chances of living longer than women with heart problems who do not take estrogens, studies indicate. However, the claim that estrogens can lower the number of heart attacks and other episodes by up to 80 percent, as some research has put forth, needs further validation.

If you have a history of thrombosis (an abnormal blood condition that promotes blood clotting), most doctors traditionally would advise against estrogens, given the past association between blood clotting and the birth control pill's high estrogen doses. Yet some physicians are revising their recommendations in light of recent data that indicate that today's lower doses of estrogens no longer appear to pose a threat for *pulmonary embolism* (a blood clot to the lungs) or *thrombophlebitis* (the inflammation of a vein, often in conjunction with a blood clot). The three-year PEPI trial brought more positive news: Levels of *fibrinogen,* a blood-clot-forming protein, stayed fairly stable in the study's HRT users compared to nonusers. Since your body produces more fibrinogen as you age, this suggests that HRT might help cap that rise.

Some doctors now maintain that if you've shown no sign of thrombosis in the last two to four years, estrogen therapy not only may be safe for you, but may even help to guard against recurrences of clotting. To be on the safe side, a physician may recommend a nonoral route of therapy, such as transdermal estrogens, in order to guard against liver stimulation and an increase in blood-clotting factors.

The Cardiovascular Effects of Progestins and Androgens

If your HRT regimen includes both estrogens and progestins, the cardiovascular effects of prescribed estrogens are just part of the story. An equally important consideration is: What do progestins do to the circulatory system?

Compared to the limited amount researchers know about estrogens' interaction with the heart and circulatory system, even less is known about the impact of progestins. Unfortunately, even the bits and pieces that we do know are controversial. Some research has suggested that progestins, when added to estrogens, can lower the levels of HDL, the "good" cholesterol that estrogens enhance. Theoretically, progestins may counteract estrogen's beneficial widening of the coronary arteries. Other research doesn't support that conclusion, especially those investigations that studied the newer, purer progestins. Further complicating the picture is recent evidence that while supplemental progestins may reduce HDL levels for some months, blood cholesterol levels aren't adversely affected by longer-term therapy.

What many researchers seem to agree on is that certain types of progestins and higher dosages may reduce estrogen's benefits to cholesterol levels more than other types of progestins. The *C-19 progestins*—a class of progestins that have androgenlike properties—appear to have more adverse effects than *C-21 progestins,* which are less androgenic. Medroxyprogesterone acetate (MPA), the most commonly prescribed progestin in the United States, is one type of C-21 progestin.

Unlike certain synthetic progestins, natural progesterone doesn't seem to affect blood cholesterol one way or the other. However, in addition to its high cost, oral natural progesterone can cause sedativelike side effects. Moreover, when it crosses the liver, it's broken down to such an extent that it no longer resembles the pure progesterone produced by the ovaries. For these reasons, oral progesterone hasn't been commonly used.

Until recently, a different form of natural progesterone—micronized oral progesterone—wasn't that widely used or available. However, that might change. Recent findings from the PEPI trial showed that micronized (natural) progesterone, when combined with conjugated equine estrogens (CEE), had less of a blunting effect on estrogen-boosted HDL, the "good" cholesterol, than did the synthetic progestin medroxyprogesterone acetate (MPA). CEEs plus micronized progesterone produced HDL levels that were nearly as high as when CEEs were taken alone.

Progesterone is also available in suppository form. However, since suppository medication can leak out the vagina, some women find this approach inconvenient. Suppositories can also interfere with sexual activity.

Until synthetic progestins' influence on blood lipoproteins is better understood, should you worry about their effects on your heart health? Judging from current research, no. Estrogens' beneficial effects on blood cholesterol levels appear to override any negative effects from progestins—if indeed progestins affect blood cholesterol at all. Research indicates that postmenopausal women on a progestin-estrogen regimen still receive more heart protection than women not on replacement therapy. Using a C-21 progestin such as medroxyprogesterone acetate at the lowest effective dose can help ensure that the progestins you're taking aren't undermining the cardiac protection provided by estrogens.

As regards supplemental androgens, older studies have raised concerns that these hormones can adversely affect blood cholesterol. However, research into newer combinations and doses of androgens and estrogens has shown no significant impact on triglyceride, HDL, or LDL levels. It remains unclear what role androgens may play in other features of heart health.

MEDICATION TIPS

• A dose of 0.625 mg/day of oral conjugated equine estrogens or an equivalent dose of a different type estrogen may provide protection from heart disease and may effectively treat a range of circulatory disorders. However, more than 1.25 mg/day may have adverse effects on the circulatory system.

• If your uterus is intact and your doctor has prescribed estrogens for their heart-protective qualities, he or she will probably also prescribe progestins for endometrial protection. Results from the PEPI trial indicate that micronized progesterone may be the progestin that least blocks estrogens' HDL benefits.

• Although estrogens lack FDA approval for the treatment of heart disease, doctors regularly prescribe them for that purpose.

Hormone Therapy and Osteoporosis

As far back as the 1940s, the prominent MGH endocrinologist Fuller Albright observed that when women's hormone levels fall after menopause, the loss of bone mass accelerates and can hasten osteoporosis. It wasn't until the late 1970s, however, that new methods for measuring bone helped support the premise that if you put estrogen back into a woman's system after menopause, it can slow bone deterioration. By now, the bone-related benefits of estrogens are well known to physicians, who often recommend estrogens as the first choice of treatment for known or suspected bone loss. (Exogenous estrogens and calcitonin are the only two medications currently approved by the FDA for the treatment of bone loss, but newer agents will also soon be approved.) It's estimated that an 80-year-

"I went on HRT twenty-five years ago because of a serious family history of osteoporosis," recounts a 70-year-old doctor of internal medicine. "My mother and two maternal aunts all suffered from osteoporosis. There's no question in my mind that estrogen has helped my bones. I haven't shrunk like my mother did, and there's no indication of osteoporosis. I plan to continue therapy until the day I die, unless a contraindication like cancer arises."

old woman who has taken estrogens since menopause will lose only 10 percent of her bone density, compared to the 30 percent lost by an 80-year-old woman who has never used estrogens.

If you're taking estrogens to treat bone loss, don't expect the therapy to significantly *reverse* bone loss. Estrogens can't cure osteoporosis, nor can any other known treatment. Any increase in bone density as a result of estrogen therapy is nominal. Instead, estrogens primarily *retard* bone loss and preserve existing bone. (Since no current treatment significantly stimulates bone growth, there's all the more reason for middle-aged women to maintain healthy bone through nutrition, exercise, and other healthful habits.)

Women mistakenly believe that if they take estrogens for the short haul—while they're in their fifties, say—they will significantly lower their chances for fracture in their seventies or eighties, when fractures are most prevalent. In fact, however, the risk for fracture in later age appears best averted through longer-lasting estrogen therapy.

Studies have shown that for the first five to seven years after menopause, bone density decreases at an accelerated rate. Therefore, if you're at risk for osteoporosis, you might want to consider hormone replacement or an alternative treatment as soon as possible after a natural or surgical menopause.

Findings from the Framingham Study published in *The New England Journal of Medicine* in 1993 concluded that at least seven years of estrogen therapy are needed to have a prolonged effect on bone, and therapy for even this length may not stave off fracture in women age 75 and older. The data suggested that estrogens' therapeutic effects wear off soon after therapy is discontinued, even when estrogens were taken for ten or more years. When estrogens are stopped, bone density can decrease as rapidly as seen directly after menopause. "Among the women 75 years old and older, the effect of prolonged therapy [ten or more years] was slight," the research team reported. However, this study and many others stress that it's never too late to start estrogen replacement. Begun late in life, it can still inhibit bone loss to some extent.

The Framingham data prompted a *NEJM* editorial by menopause authorities Drs. Bruce Ettinger and Deborah Grady, who had this to say: "To provide maximal protection, estrogen treatment may have to be started at the time of the menopause and never stopped." The resulting "improvement in bone density is likely to reduce the risk of fracture by about two-thirds, but having to take estrogen for the rest of one's life reduces the appeal of this preventive strategy."

Since most people find it hard to stick with even short-term medication schedules, taking HRT for twenty to forty years seems unrealistic unless the method of administration makes compliance especially easy. More important, although very long-term estrogen use may benefit bone, other cell types and systems may react adversely if exposed to estrogens indefinitely.

The Effects of Progestins and Androgens on Bone Loss

Along with estrogens, there's evidence that progestins also work on bone's behalf. But because it takes such large amounts of exogenous progestins to reduce bone loss—amounts that reportedly may have a negative impact on blood cholesterol—they are seldom used as a primary treatment for deteriorating bone. When standard doses are combined with estrogens to thwart endometrial overgrowth, the combination may work synergistically to preserve bone density, some studies suggest.

Androgens are well-known enhancers of bone and muscle growth. But they haven't been specifically enlisted for bone therapy, since past studies have raised questions about their effects on blood cholesterol. Moreover, the more potent doses needed for this therapy are more likely to produce masculinizing side effects. Newer research into the relationship between standard doses of androgens and blood lipoproteins shows no serious detrimental effects on blood cholesterol. How much do the small amounts of androgens added to HRT regimens for the purpose of treating libido actually help stabilize bone? One new study suggests that estrogen-androgen combinations may indeed benefit bone density, yet may not have the same good effect on cholesterol levels as estrogens taken alone.

MEDICATION TIPS
• A dose of 0.5 mg/day of oral estradiol works to help prevent bone loss. With the skin patch, an even lower estradiol dose works: 0.05 mg/day. Because the patch's medication doesn't make a first pass through the liver, as do oral estrogens, less medication is broken down and lost. Hence, a lower transdermal dose can be as effective as a higher orally administered dose. In many of the stud-

ies that show the effectiveness of these dosages for bone, the study participants also took calcium.

• It's been found that although 0.3 mg/day of oral conjugated equine estrogens may not be enough for bone therapy, a dose of 1.25 mg/day is more than enough. However, 0.3 mg/day may suffice if you also take calcium supplements. The standard oral dose of 0.625 mg/day CEE or an equivalent dose of a different oral estrogen is considered efficient to retard the bone loss seen in the years immediately following menopause.

• If, upon menopause, a bone densitometry measurement reveals that you're at a higher-than-normal risk for osteoporotic fractures, you may want to consider estrogen replacement for at least seven to ten years.

• If your uterus is intact and you're taking estrogens to retard bone loss, it's likely that your doctor will also prescribe progestins for endometrial protection. Some studies suggest that progestins, when added to estrogens, may also help protect bone.

Hormone Therapy and Hot Flashes

Postmenopausal Treatment

In some 95 percent of cases, estrogen replacement diminishes the hot flashes caused by ovarian failure to the point where they usually stop for the duration of treatment. Estrogens are widely considered the most effective form of therapy for menopausal hot flashes. However, if you have a medical condition that prohibits estrogen use or if you prefer nonhormonal treatment, other approaches that include alternatives to drugs are available. (See Section Three.)

If you're using HRT to control hot flashes, don't expect

immediate relief. Usually it takes a minimum of two to four weeks of treatment before your hot flashes will begin to subside significantly. You should also realize that if you stop treatment abruptly, your hot flashes can return—possibly within a week or two. If you intend to halt treatment, it's important that you wean your body of supplemental estrogens very gradually. For example, reduce your intake from seven to six pills per week for a month, then five pills per week for a month, and so on. If you're using the transdermal delivery system, remove the patch a day earlier per week for a month, then two days earlier for the next month and so on. You should continue the usual dose of progestins until you've completely weaned yourself off estrogens. No ill effects will occur when you abruptly stop progestins.

If you withdraw estrogens gradually but your hot flashes nevertheless return and prove bothersome or severe, you may need to go back on estrogens.

Perimenopausal Treatment

If you have disruptive hot flashes before menopause, most doctors recommend that you hold off on standard postmenopausal hormone doses and consider using a low-dose oral contraceptive (OC) pill instead—as long as you don't smoke or have a health disorder that prevents you from using the Pill. The Pill's estrogen and progestin content will relieve your hot flashes, regulate your menstrual cycle, and stem the irregular bleeding that occurs during perimenopause. As discussed, the amounts of estrogen in the low-dose pill are actually more potent than the dose of 0.625 mg of CEE commonly used for replacement therapy after menopause.

If you were to take the 0.625 mg dose of CEE before

menopause, you would probably experience "withdrawal" bleeding on top of your irregular menstrual bleeding, which you might find disruptive and annoying. If you take the low-dose pill, because of its higher estrogen-progestin content you'll experience only regulated menstrual bleeding. You and your doctor should aim for the Pill with the lowest effective dose.

Be aware that OCs will mask menopause; your menstrual cycles will keep coming, even when menopause shuts down the internal hormones that normally produce menstruation. Although not always foolproof, a simple blood test that measures follicle-stimulating hormone (FSH) levels can tell you if menopause has taken place. To get an accurate FSH reading, many physicians recommend that you stop taking OCs a few weeks before you take an FSH test.

Since a low-dose OC is more potent than HRT replacement doses given after menopause, it carries more contraindications. Your doctor may advise against the Pill if you smoke or have any of the following conditions: diabetes, hypertension, breast cancer, pregnancy, liver disease, irregular bleeding, a history of blood clotting, or heart disease.

When used to combat perimenopausal hot flashes, the Pill has the added benefit of providing contraception. During this midpoint in their lives, many women mistakenly think they won't get pregnant and take fewer birth control precautions.

Progestins and Androgens for Hot Flashes

For those of you plagued by hot flashes after menopause but unable to use estrogens because of a medical condition, replacement progestins offer a useful alternative.

(Their use during perimenopause as a hot-flash reliever hasn't been studied.) Progestins are capable of quelling hot flashes in 70 percent of cases. A potential drawback, however, is their disruptive side effects—irritability, mood swings, and breast tenderness—to which some women are more susceptible to than others. If, in particular, you're concerned about estrogens' impact on breast cancer, you may want to look into progestins for postmenopausal hot-flash relief. Research has uncovered no signs that progestins increase the risk of breast cancer.

While androgens taken alone haven't been reported to bring hot-flash relief, it's suspected (but not solidly proven) that androgens in combination with estrogens can be more effective in quelling hot flashes than estrogens alone.

MEDICATION TIPS

• If your perimenopausal hot flashes are so disruptive that you want to treat them, doctors will usually prescribe a low-dose contraceptive pill. Most utilize one of two different estrogen bases—ethinyl estradiol and mestranol—which are equally effective.

• For the treatment of postmenopausal hot flashes, physicians generally prescribe a dose in the range of 0.3 to 1.25 mg/day of oral conjugated equine estrogens or equivalent doses of other estrogens.

• If your uterus is intact and you're taking estrogens, your doctor will likely prescribe progestins as well, in order to counteract any possibility of endometrial disorders.

• If progestins are your primary treatment for hot flashes, your physician will likely recommend 10 mg/day of medroxyprogesterone acetate or 20 mg/twice a day of megestrol acetate. This latter progestin has been found to reduce the frequency of hot flashes by 50 percent.

• If an estrogen dosage isn't quelling hot flashes and the dosage is increased, as long as a protective dosage of progestins is in use for endometrial purposes, usually that dosage can stay the same. Bear in mind that if estrogen isn't working, it can mean that your hot flashes are being caused by an overactive thyroid gland, not estrogen loss.

Hormone Therapy and Fatal Colon Cancer

A recently reported study by American Cancer Society researchers has added weight to what several smaller studies previously have found: Estrogen therapy appears to lower the risk of fatal colon cancer in postmenopausal women. In the ACS study, all current users of estrogen had a 45 percent risk reduction compared to nonusers; former users had a 19 percent risk reduction. For current users who had been on estrogen for ten or more years, there was a 55 percent reduction in risk of colon cancer deaths. Current use (versus former use) and longer use (versus shorter use) lowered the risk the most.

More research is needed to further substantiate these findings, as well as investigate whatever explanations lie behind them. Scientists so far have discovered that estrogen bears the ability of reducing bile acids in the colon that promote tumors. But there may be other contributing factors as well.

Hormone Therapy and
Vaginal Disorders

Oral and nonoral estrogens can effectively revitalize vaginal lubrication, thereby reducing vaginal dryness. If you're looking to relieve vaginal dryness alone, your doctor may recommend a vaginal estrogen cream. Vaginal creams tend to be more effective at treating the vagina directly than nonvaginal estrogen treatments. But even with the use of an estrogen cream, you may find it takes several weeks before treatment starts alleviating symptoms. Estrogens first have to build up the cellular components that help restore moistness. The results can be worth waiting for as most women—even older women—experience a definite improvement in vaginal tissue.

> "About six years after I'd gone through menopause, it [vaginal dryness] was so bad, I didn't feel like having sex with my husband. I was using everything short of motor oil and nothing worked. My doctor began me on vaginal estrogen creams. By the second month, there was noticeable improvement."

Few studies have determined replacement estrogens' effects on other postmenopausal urogenital problems. However, limited research indicates that estrogens can help prevent urinary tract infections and may possibly improve certain kinds of incontinence.

In an analysis of studies devoted to urinary incontinence in postmenopausal women and published in the journal *Obstetrics and Gynecology,* researchers found that "estrogen subjectively improves urinary incontinence," meaning that the women studied felt that their incontinence had lessened with estrogen therapy. However, in several individual studies of stress incontinence (urinary leakage that occurs with a sneeze or heavy lifting), estrogen therapy didn't appear to bring improvement. Until further investigation unfolds, it's hard to know exactly to what degree estrogens can restore bladder control.

In 1993 *The New England Journal of Medicine* carried encouraging news of vaginal estrogens' positive impact on urinary tract infections (UTIs). A study of 93 postmenopausal women with a history of recurrent UTIs suggested that infections among women who used a vaginal estrogen cream were significantly reduced compared to women given a placebo, or inert medication. Many more of the estrogen users, as compared to nonusers, remained free of UTIs, the scientists reported. Estrogen users experienced only 0.5 episodes of infection in contrast to 5.9 for the placebo group. Estrogen use was thought to restore adequate levels of acidity in the vagina and encourage the presence of beneficial bacteria (lactobacilli). Both these conditions help ward off the less desirable bacteria that are associated with urinary tract infections. The researchers suggest that vaginal estrogen creams may be used as an alternative to long-term preventive antibiotics

---

"Shortly after menopause, I started getting a burning sensation when I urinated. I thought it might just go away so I didn't do anything about it. Not long after, I went on estrogens [oral 0.625 CEE] and progestins for bone protection, and within a few weeks the burning went away. My doctor explained that lower urinary tract tissue can produce symptoms of estrogen depletion after menopause, and that my estrogen therapy must have worked to revitalize the tissue."

for urinary tract infections, especially in cases where antibiotics induce undesirable side effects.

Too little research exists to say to what degree estrogen therapy can help maintain the integrity and strength of urogenital organs, muscles, and other structural components after menopause. Yet there's evidence that its enhancement of blood flow, cell rigidity, tissue thickness, and other estrogen-dependent qualities can help preserve the structure and the function of organs.

> "I used to get a lot of bladder infections, but they cleared up once I went on estrogen."

MEDICATION TIPS

• The standard oral dose of 0.625 mg/CEE or an equivalent dose of another oral or transdermal estrogen may not effectively revitalize vaginal tissue in some women. If you're using this oral dose for other menopausal conditions, you may also need to use a vaginal cream to ease vaginal dryness.

• Although the oral dose of 0.625 mg/CEE or an oral/transdermal equivalent may not work to revitalize some women's vaginal tissue, it can work for others. In fact, even the low oral dose of 0.3 mg/day may be all some women need for vaginal recovery—a lower dose than what's normally used for treatment of hot flashes or osteoporosis. For endometrial protection, progestins usually are needed to accompany estrogen, even the low oral dose of 0.3 mg.

• Of the many different estrogen vaginal creams available, all appear to be equally effective for vaginal dryness. What might come as a surprise is the fact that varying amounts of estrogen from these preparations can be absorbed across the vagina into the bloodstream. Therefore, if your uterus is intact, your doctor very likely will prescribe intermittent progestins in conjunction with these creams to lower your risk for endometrial overgrowth. For other medication tips pertaining to vaginal estrogen creams, see Chapter 7.

• If you've been postmenopausal for twenty or more years, it's advisable to initiate treatment with low-estrogen doses on alternate days. A 70-year-old woman getting larger doses may experience breast tenderness until her tissues adjust.

Hormone Therapy, Sexual Functioning, and Responsiveness

Prescribing small amounts of androgens to women who experience diminished libido or sex drive after menopause is a fairly new practice and one that is gaining momentum. Too few studies exist to say exactly what proportion of postmenopausal women notice a downturn in sexual arousal and pleasure after surgical or natural menopause, but it appears to be a common problem. Research led by Dr. Barbara B. Sherwin, a psychologist and codirector of McGill University's Menopause Clinic, and gynecologist Dr. Morrie Gelfand, a McGill professor, has shown that an estrogen-testosterone preparation given to women after the surgical removal of the ovaries and/or uterus can renew the "mental" elements of sex—libido, arousal, fantasizing. Estrogens taken alone had a lesser effect.

These findings may tempt you to conclude that androgen therapy can serve as a panacea for postmenopausal sexual disinterest or unresponsiveness. Be aware, however, that even the researchers who reported the above results urge that androgens be used with discretion. A depressed state of mind may have little to do with hormone depletion, they caution, but a lot to do with the stresses and strains of everyday life. Furthermore, despite the observed androgen-libido link, some researchers steadfastly warn that we still don't know how closely connected androgens are to libido, and that doctors should proceed cautiously when prescribing them. Altogether, androgen therapy is more often considered for women experiencing lowered libido and depression after the surgical removal of the ovaries and uterus.

After a natural menopause, androgen therapy's use should be determined on an individual basis. It could very well be that after menopause your body will still be producing sufficient amounts of androgens, although some women produce less. Ovarian failure does away with the production of some androgens, but it does not interfere with the output of the potent hormone testosterone, which continues to be produced in residual cells of the ovary. If you're considering this therapy, also be aware that supplemental androgens can cause facial hair growth, oily skin, and acne. (Lower doses can lessen the likelihood of these and other side effects.) For years there's been concern that long-term androgen therapy can negatively alter blood cholesterol. While some research into newer, lower-dose androgen regimens hasn't found this to be true, a slight androgen-induced negative change was recently observed in one study. It's probably wisest, then, to aim for the lowest dose possible for the sake of a lesser impact on blood cholesterol.

Estrogens can also improve sexual functioning by treating symptoms like vaginal dryness. But older women in particular should realize that a gradual decline in sexual

"I used to enjoy sex so much. My husband and I had equal sex drives. At some point around menopause, I lost that feeling, so I began taking testosterone, along with estrogen and progesterone. Testosterone helps with the libido a little, but it's not the same. It makes me feel more physically aggressive in the way I handle situations."

functioning can be a normal part of aging and that estrogens aren't a cure-all for reduced sexual ability in later life.

Medication Tips

• Women have reported that a low-dose androgen (2.5 mg/day of methyltestosterone) can increase sexual desire within a month. Although androgens can be taken alone, most often they are prescribed in combination with estrogens.

• Note that even though physicians prescribe androgens for the treatment of decreased libido in women, they have not been approved by the FDA for this use.

• Because oral androgens can affect the liver, you may not be able to take them if you have a liver disorder.

Hormone Therapy and Mood

It's generally believed that sex hormones alter mood by interacting with brain neurotransmitters. Replacement hormones can sometimes improve a woman's frame of mind and mood—especially, as has been observed, after her ovaries are removed. This surgery and the resulting sudden drop in ovarian estrogens and androgens can result in depression, a diminished sense of well-being, and reduced libido.

Research undertaken by Dr. Sherwin and coworkers indicates that women who receive either estrogens or an estrogen-androgen preparation after surgical menopause feel more energetic, confident, and positive about life than those not treated. Sherwin and others have noted that the addition of androgens, rather than estrogens used alone, especially appears to improve a woman's mental state.

If you're feeling down, there are many reasons other than hormone depletion that may account for your mood. Therefore, supplemental hormones aren't necessarily going to relieve lethargy, depression, anxiety, a poor outlook, or low self-esteem. If you're considering hormones specifically for the treatment of mood disorders, a trial dose of estrogens can be a useful way of discovering if hormone depletion is at the root of your problem. Should your mental outlook improve after one to two months, you can decide to continue on hormones. If it doesn't, you might consider other options, such as counseling. If you're feeling severely depressed and suicidal, it's best to seek counseling right away. Depression can be extremely debilitating, but with the right help it can be overcome.

> "Estrogen, almost overnight, infinitely restored my sense of well-being, which took a real header right before menopause."

MEDICATION TIPS

- In certain circumstances, especially if you've had your ovaries removed, you might consider estrogens-androgens specifically to treat your mood symptoms.
- If depression appears to be associated with perimenopausal hormone changes, some doctors might try a

trial run of ERT to see if this reduces depression before psychotropic drugs are considered.

• Androgens in tandem with estrogens are available in tablets as well as injected preparations. Choose the method you find most convenient.

Hormone Therapy and Your Brain

New research holds out the possibility that estrogen therapy may help safeguard certain mental capabilities. As seen in Chapter 3, one large study of retired women in California showed a 40 percent lower incidence of Alzheimer's among estrogen users as compared to nonusers. Research also indicates that estrogens may help fortify short-term verbal memory and brain activity that affects balance and other aspects of motor coordination. There have been no findings that estrogens improve visual memory or general attention span. Since various regions of the brain also contain progesterone and androgen receptors, there's speculation that replacement therapy utilizing these hormones also may affect brain functioning.

While there are signs that estrogens may aid specific brain-related tasks, investigations to date are too prelimi-

---

"Many menopausal patients I see complain of forgetfulness—of not being able to remember names and phone numbers. They blame menopause; but their forgetfulness is probably age-related, not menopause-related. Younger women who experience a premature menopause show no such memory decline. But just like middle-aged women, middle-aged men also complain of memory loss—yet they can't use menopause as an excuse!"

nary to act upon. At this stage in the research it's not recommended that newly menopausal women rush out and take estrogens solely for the purpose of brain-cell protection. Estrogen depletion certainly doesn't translate into instant dementia, nor is there conclusive proof that it can contribute to cognitive disabilities decades later. If you're taking estrogen supplements for a particular health reason and it becomes more firmly proven that estrogens do in fact benefit brain functioning, so much the better.

Hormone Therapy and Your Skin

Because supplemental hormones can provide many health benefits, it's easy to forget that they are potent drugs with risks and side effects. Taking hormones simply for skin care is like taking a massive dose of antibiotics for a small cut on the finger. You may not like the wrinkling, thinning, or dryness of skin that comes with age, but these conditions aren't life-threatening or physically impairing. Therefore, most doctors don't recommend HRT solely for skin care. If, on the other hand, your skin shows marked signs of postmenopausal deterioration and is very dry or chapped or easily cut or bruised, your doctor—depending upon his or her viewpoint—might recommend estrogen therapy. Be aware, however, that exogenous estrogens' ability to relieve such skin conditions hasn't been proven. Moreover, HRT is not a miracle anti-aging formula.

There is clear evidence that HRT can alter the skin. But the extent of its benefits for skin changed by sun exposure, aging, and smoking is unclear. In what its authors describe as "the first randomized, double-blind, placebo-controlled study addressing the effects of estrogen replacement therapy on skin thickness," a 1994 Canadian study evaluated

60 postmenopausal nuns (ages 51 to 71) whose limited exposure to sun and smoking provided a clearer reading of what changing hormone levels, without confounding factors, do to skin. After twelve months of taking standard doses of oral estrogens, those in the treated group showed a 30 percent increase in dermis (the inner layer of skin) thickness and a 11.5 percent increase in overall skin thickness. No significant skin changes were observed in the placebo group.

Since the 1950s, evidence has been accumulating that replacement estrogens, sometimes in combination with testosterone, can restore or maintain skin thickness and skin collagen. There are also claims that estrogens can reverse the dry, flaky, easily bruised skin seen after menopause. However, other studies have failed to report a correlation between estrogen use and improved skin.

What's accepted is that during the years immediately following menopause, postmenopausal skin collagen loss appears to parallel bone loss. Collagen loss accelerates during the first several years after menopause, whereas skin thickness wanes more gradually. This would suggest that if supplemental estrogens do indeed benefit skin, starting them soon after menopause might help protect against this fall-off in collagen.

Some research has found that estrogens can inhibit the loss of skin collagen and thickness within six months, and even restore some of what's lost. (Again, bear in mind that other studies have found no improvement.) There is also some indication that as skin thickness increases, wrinkling might be reduced. On the other hand, estrogens don't appear to return skin's elasticity, according to Dr. George S. Richardson, associate chief of MGH's Vincent OB-GYN Service. Moreover, once a certain threshold of improvement is reached, long-term hormone use does not appear to have a further effect on skin.

The point is that estrogens' effect on skin is still unproven, so it should not be a deciding factor as you weigh taking HRT. If you go on hormones and see some skin improvement, consider it a happy side effect. In the meantime, protecting your skin against the sun's harmful rays and not smoking are the best proven ways to help your skin.

Can Hormone Therapy Help You Live Longer?

Increasingly, researchers are looking at the overall impact of hormone therapy on the quality and length of a woman's life. Their findings indicate that women who use estrogen for longer than seven years generally have less disease and may live longer. Much of this research, however, involves only the use of oral estrogens, so researchers don't have a clear picture of how nonoral estrogens, progestins, and androgens further impact disease-related mortality. Also, since many of those studied tend to be women who look after themselves and their health, they may be generally healthier and more disease-free than most women.

Drawing from a prospective study of postmenopausal women residing in a California retirement community, researchers reported that after 7.5 years, women using oral conjugated estrogens had a 20 percent lower death rate from all causes than women not on hormones. After fifteen years of replacement therapy, women who were still using estrogens had a 40 percent lower death rate—regardless of whether they were taking a high dose (1.25 mg daily) or a low dose (0.625 mg daily).

In a very different type of study, a group of researchers used established data to make educated projections about the possible health benefits and risks for a hypothetical group of 10,000 women (age 50 to 75) taking estrogens for twenty-five years compared to another hypothetical group of 10,000 women not on estrogens. The researchers projected that the estrogen-taking group would have 567 fewer fatal heart disease events (48 percent) and 75 fewer deaths (49 percent) from complications of hip fractures compared to the nonusers. However, the estrogen users would also experience 39 additional deaths from breast cancer (a 21 percent increase) and 29 additional deaths (a 207 percent increase) from endometrial cancer. This large percent increase reflects endometrial cancer's relatively low death rate to begin with: 2.6 in 100,000. (If breast cancer is diagnosed while the patient is on estrogen, it is a less fatal type of breast cancer than those found in women not on estrogens. Not that this is any compensation; any form of breast cancer can be devastating. It's also worth noting that endometrial cancer can be successfully treated if detected in its earliest stages. But most important of all is the fact that women can avoid the estrogen-induced increased risk of endometrial cancer by taking estrogen-progestin combinations.)

When researchers weighed the hypothetical lives saved through estrogens' reduction of heart disease against the other risks, they felt that the risks were more than offset by the benefits of estrogen replacement therapy.

Despite the researchers' optimism, it should be noted that estrogen therapy's protectiveness against bone fracture would most likely pay off at a later age, while its added risk for breast cancer could surface at a younger age. A study released in 1996 suggested that estrogens are associated with an increase in longevity. However, before you leap to the conclusion that estrogens are the fountain of youth, you should recognize that the study indicated a significant increase in longevity only for women older than seventy. That means that you would have to take hormones for at least fifteen years before seeing a positive effect on heart disease. Of course, you would have to balance this benefit against any potential risks that may occur at a younger age. Further, this study was not a randomized trial; it's possible that women who are compliant and take medications are simply more likely to live longer than those who don't. When deciding whether to take a hormone, you should therefore take into account that while it could be beneficial at one age, it might be risky at another. Now let's talk more about these risks.

Risks Associated with Hormone Therapy

The previous chapter listed those medical conditions that can raise a red flag against estrogen use. Below is a more thorough discussion of those conditions. Since most women's greatest concern is estrogen replacement's association with endometrial cancer and breast cancer. Those specific issues are discussed in length later in this chapter.

The medical conditions that may present roadblocks to ERT include:

Cancer

If you have ever had any malignancies associated with estrogen-sensitive cells in your breast or uterus, or any susceptibility to tumor formation, you will probably be strongly advised against estrogen therapy. If you have a strong family history of estrogen-related cancers, the same caution applies.

In May of 1995, a study done by the American Cancer Society reported that, among those evaluated, women who had been on estrogen therapy for eleven years or more showed a 70 percent increased risk for fatal ovarian cancer compared to nonusers. The increased risk for those who used estrogen for shorter durations wasn't deemed significant. While these new findings might seem cause for alarm, people should realize they are far from conclusive. "This is not definitive. This is only one study. There are others that don't suggest an increased risk, and still others that show that estrogen therapy has a protective effect on ovarian cancer," says Eugenia E. Calle, Director of Analytic Epidemiology for the American Cancer Society. "The 70 percent doesn't necessarily reflect reality. Much more research is required for a broader consensus."

Because the numbers of women normally afflicted by ovarian cancer are low—in comparison, say, to breast cancer—if a 70 percent increased risk did prove realistic, such an increase reflects relatively few additional ovarian-cancer deaths. (One out of 65 women will develop ovarian cancer over a lifetime; 1 in 9 will be afflicted by breast cancer.) Which is not to say, however, that any increase is acceptable. As it stands, the whole area of HRT's effect on ovarian cancer requires much more reliable measurement.

Liver Disease

If you have chronic or active liver disease (for example, hepatitis, cirrhosis, or bile problems), your doctor may well rule out estrogens, specifically estrogens in pill form. That's because after they go through the digestive tract,

"Even though I have hepatitis B, I'm using the estrogen patch—because of hot flashes and because I want its protectiveness for the heart since my menopause came a few years early—at age 47. When I first went on the patch, I had a liver profile every few months, to make sure the estrogen wasn't taxing my liver. There were no signs it was, so now I just have a liver profile once a year. A liver profile doesn't take long; it just requires getting blood drawn. Because I've experienced a small decline in sex drive, I asked my doctor about going on testosterone too, but he doesn't want me to. He feels that estrogen plus testosterone would be stretching it, in terms of possibly putting too much strain on the liver."

oral estrogens make a "first pass" through the liver, and the resulting metabolic activity can exacerbate liver ailments. Oral "micronized" estrogens, which the body can absorb more readily, can also intensify liver conditions, as can androgens and progestins. Some women with a history of liver disease may be able to take nonorally administered hormones such as the estrogen skin patch or injected hormones, depending upon the severity of their condition. Bypassing the intestinal tract, these routes avoid a "first pass" through the liver.

Gallbladder Disease

Several studies have found that postmenopausal women who take estrogens have up to a 2.5 (150 percent) increased risk of gallbladder disease. However, other research has found no increased risk.

Data from the Nurses' Health Study determined that the longer women took estrogen and the higher their dosages, the higher their risk for *cholecystectomy*, the removal of the gallbladder due to an associated malady, usually gallstones. Women studied who were currently taking hormones, mostly unopposed oral conjugated estrogens, had a 40 percent higher risk of diagnosed gallstones. However, some of this increase may represent an increased rate of diagnosis of asymptomatic gallstones, since women on estrogens generally tend to visit their doctors more often than nonusers, upping the chances that any complications will be spotted.

If you're susceptible to gallstones, estrogen therapy probably isn't right for you, since it's thought to encourage a "thickening" of bile, which results in the formation of stones. If you have no known pattern of gallbladder disease, the increased risk conferred by hormones isn't considered great enough to warn against estrogen therapy. Moreover, estrogens' associated gallbladder risk is considered fairly minimal compared to estrogens' beneficial effects.

Other Associated Risks

If you have any past or present evidence of abnormal uterine bleeding, fibroids, endometriosis, diabetes, high levels of blood cholesterol, a history of blood clots, or high blood pressure, your physician will want to thoroughly evaluate these conditions before prescribing supplemental hormones. The appropriateness of hormone therapy often depends upon the seriousness of the condition. If you have smaller fibroids that are symptom-free, for instance, you may still be able to use estrogens, since today's relatively low doses of estrogen often don't stimulate fibroid growth. On the other hand, your doctor may recommend against estrogens as a precautionary measure if you have large symptomatic fibroids. (It's possible for supplemental estrogens to cause fibroid growth even though standard estrogen doses usually don't.)

In the past, doctors have recommended against hormones for any women with a history of either thrombosis or high blood pressure. But that approach is changing. If you had either of these conditions long ago, using estrogens now might not only be safe but even beneficial, given estrogens' heart protection.

Hormone Therapy and the Risk for Endometrial Cancer

If you have an intact uterus and decide on hormone replacement therapy in your postmenopausal years, your basic treatment will likely consist of a combination of estrogens and progestins. Estrogens represent hormone replacement's core drug, and progestins counteract the threat of endometrial cancer posed by estrogen.

Since the 1970s, numerous studies have concluded that unopposed estrogens (those given alone, without progestins) are associated with a sizable increase in the risk of *endometrial hyperplasia,* a proliferation of cells that sometimes results in cancer. It's been found that 30 percent of women taking unopposed conjugated estrogens (0.625 mg daily for 25 of 30 days each month) develop hyperplasia after one year. While this may seem a high percentage, as few as 1 to 3 percent of untreated cases of hyperplasia are thought to progress into malignancies. Nonetheless, since it's now known that this risk can be countered with the addition of progestins, the estrogen-progestin combination is frequently considered the prudent choice to minimize the possibility of cancer. As it turns out, this regimen isn't only precautionary: It also can be preventive. Research indicates that postmenopausal women taking estrogens in tandem with certain progestins (notably, norethindrone or medroxyprogesterone) have a lower incidence of uterine cancer than women who take no hormones at all.

Physicians commonly recommend adding progestins for a minimum of ten days to each month's intake of estrogens. However, if you're using a dose of 0.625 mg/day of conjugated estrogens and cannot tolerate the side effects of progestins, which include mood shifts and breast tenderness, the threat of hyperplasia is so minimal that you can probably take progestins for seven to nine days and still get the protection you need.

If you opt for unopposed low-dose estrogens—for the relief of short-term menopausal symptoms or because progestins' side effects prove too onerous—you need to be aware of the possibility of hyperplasia and how to manage that risk. You should have periodic endometrial evaluations to measure the growth of the endometrium lining and detect the early warning signs of any overgrowth. An increasingly used technique called *transvaginal ultrasound* provides a convenient way of measuring the lining's thickness. When employing this painless procedure, which takes only a few minutes, a physician inserts a probe into the vagina that transmits a view of the uterine cavity and ovaries to a nearby monitor. A full bladder isn't required as it is for an abdominal ultrasound.

If this approach shows the endometrium is more than 4 mm thick, your physician might consider a biopsy—a sampling of endometrial tissue to screen for possible cancer. In a biopsy, which can be somewhat painful, the physician uses a catheter inserted into the uterine cavity to extract a small portion of uterine lining. If analysis of the tissue shows you have excess endometrial growth, you'll need to add progestins to your regimen or stop estrogen therapy.

If your uterus is intact and you're using unopposed estrogens, schedule an endometrial evaluation at least once a year, every year. I personally recommend you have endometrial testing every six months for the first two years after you start ERT. (The impetus behind this suggestion is not based on firm data, just commonsense caution.) If your endometrial growth remains normal, you can then scale back evaluations to once a year. A convenient schedule might be:

six months after starting ERT . . . . ultrasound
twelve months . . . . biopsy
eighteen months . . . . ultrasound
twenty-four months . . . . biopsy

Medication Tips

• It's not known how low a dose of progestins can safely lower the risk of endometrial overgrowth incurred by unopposed estrogens. Currently, an oral dose of 5 mg medroxyprogesterone acetate added to estrogens for seven to ten days each month is thought to be adequate coverage. (This presents a 1 to 3 percent risk of hyperplasia.) I often start my patients on a dose of 10 mg/day/MPA for thirteen days a month. This leaves room for dropping to a lower dose if a patient experiences unwanted side effects, since doses as low as 2.5 mg/day/MPA for thirteen days a month appear to provide endometrial protection. (Thirteen days of progestins almost always cancel out any risk of hyperplasia.)

Hormone Therapy and the Risk for Breast Cancer

Will the estrogens used in hormone replacement therapy increase your chances of developing breast cancer in your postmenopausal years? In any review of HRT's risks and benefits, no other question has elicited so much debate and concern—debate sparked by an array of conflicting findings and concern heightened by breast cancer's increased prevalence during this century.

Here's my short answer: After seven to ten years of exogenous estrogen use after age fifty, some postmenopausal women do show a distinct increased risk in breast cancer compared to women not on estrogens. We don't know why; it could be that some women are more susceptible to breast cancer than others. Several recent analyses of studies concerned with hormone therapy and breast cancer confirm this higher risk rate. An overview performed by the Centers for Disease Control, for instance, showed that fifteen-year users of estrogens had an average 30 percent increased risk for breast cancer compared to nonusers. Women who used estrogens for up to five years did not appear to have an additional risk.

In a report from the Nurses' Health Study, recently published in *The New England Journal of Medicine,* data showed that five or more years of hormone replacement therapy was associated with a 30 to 40 percent increase in breast cancer incidence compared to when HRT was never used. A few weeks later, another study conducted by researchers at the University of Washington found that women who used combined progestin-estrogen therapy for up to eight years didn't appear to face an increased risk. These back-to-back findings lent to confusion. Yet what the particulars of these and other studies suggest is that longer-term HRT poses a greater risk for breast cancer than shorter-term HRT.

"The literature in general supports an association of an approximately 30 to 50 percent increased risk after long-term estrogen use of fifteen to twenty years," notes Eugenia E. Calle, of the American Cancer Society.

To really understand what a 30 to 50 percent increased risk means, one has to first look at the incidence rate for breast cancer among all women—a rate that increases noticeably with age, especially after age 50. According to 1986–1990 figures compiled by the National Cancer Institute, women aged 30 to 34 face an annual incidence rate of 26.6 cases of breast cancer per 100,000 women. For women aged 55 to 59, this rate increases to 274 per 100,000. By ages 65 to 69, the incidence rate is 411 cases per 100,000 women. Therefore, when we talk about a 50 percent increased rate for a 68-year-old woman who's taken estrogens for fifteen years, this translates into an incidence rate of up to 617 in 100,000 versus the 411 per 100,000 for a 68-year-old nonuser. This amounts to an increased risk of 2 in 1000. As small a risk as this may seem, if you develop breast cancer, the experience can be devastating. Even a small added risk can be unacceptable.

Throughout your lifetime at any given age, you never face an incidence rate of greater than 1 in 200. The oft-quoted statistic that a woman has a 1-in-9 chance of developing breast cancer is misleading, since these figures refer to the cumulative probability of developing breast cancer over a lifetime (from birth to age 85) and not to the risk encountered at any given age.

According to 1991 figures released by the National Center for Health Statistics, heart disease—the leading cause of death among women—was responsible for 36 percent of fatalities; breast cancer for 5 percent. Because of the much greater protection against heart disease and osteoporosis afforded by ERT compared to the added risk of breast cancer, many health professionals believe that, for appropriate candidates, estrogen therapy is worth the risk for the sake of the benefits.

But again, the decision to take hormones comes down to a deeply personal choice, one you'll make depending on your own health profile.

There is reason to suspect that some women, apart from those with a known inherited risk, may be more prone to breast cancer after long-term estrogen use than others. Perhaps estrogens don't necessarily initiate breast cancer, but aggravate an age-related or genetically predetermined cellular defect that can lead to this cancer. Moreover, as discussed in Chapter 1, several other factors—including environmental sources and diet—may compound the unwanted effects of estrogen on breast tissue. Until we know more about the factors that promote susceptibility, every woman must weigh the benefits against the risks. If you've previously suffered a heart attack, you might opt for long-term estrogen therapy for its cardiac benefits, despite the added risk for breast cancer. If you have a family history of breast cancer, you might feel you're better off without estrogens.

In 1940 the cumulative probability over a woman's lifetime of getting breast cancer was 1 in 20 compared to 1 in 9 today. Some of the recent rise in incidence is thought to be due to the greater number of cases detected through mammography as well as women's increasing longevity, hence their increased vulnerability to breast cancer. But concern has been voiced that the rise in the incidence of breast cancer is also connected to the new trend of hormone replacement. However, only an estimated 20 to 30 percent of American women take hormones, and among those, many stop replacement therapy after a few years. Moreover, according to the American Cancer Society, the incidence of breast cancer has leveled off since 1987, while the trend toward hormone replacement has grown. It's unlikely then that exogenous hormones figure largely in the current "1-in-9" risk rate.

What can't be ignored is research showing that estrogens—both ovarian-produced and exogenous—can adversely affect breast tissue in certain situations. An early menarche and a late menopause have been associated with a greater risk for breast cancer. Researchers speculate that both these scenarios increase breast tissue's exposure to circulating estrogen and raise the possibility of tissue overgrowth, which can lead to cancer. A new study indicates that menstrual cycles that are shorter or longer than average also can heighten the risk for breast cancer. As for women under 40 who have had both ovaries removed, they have a substantially lower rate of breast cancer, perhaps because their breast tissue is no longer exposed to natural estrogen.

To sum up what the findings suggest, overexposure to estrogens may be detrimental for some women. If you opt to go on hormone therapy but have concerns about breast cancer, pay careful attention to your HRT dosage and the duration of therapy. A dose of 0.625 mg/day/CEE may be a safer route than a dose of 1.25 mg or greater. If you've taken estrogens for longer than seven to ten years since a natural menopause, you should consider a reevaluation at the end of that period. Do you have bone or heart problems that could benefit from continued estrogen use? If not, your decision whether to continue ERT could depend upon how your overall health has been affected by estrogen therapy thus far. If, on the other hand, you underwent a surgical menopause at an early age, you might more easily decide upon a longer use of replacement estrogens, since they were replacing premenopausal estrogens when you first took them.

HRT and a Family History of Breast Cancer

If you have a family history of breast cancer, even short-term replacement therapy may seem unacceptable. Research has found that a family susceptibility to this cancer places estrogen users at a 1.5 times greater risk rate for the disease than those whose families have no such history. This again suggests that some women's tissue may be genetically more vulnerable to estrogen than others.

Studies that have found an increased risk for breast cancer have also found that it may not be as lethal a cancer as in women who develop breast cancer who are not on estrogens. For example, a 1989 study from Sweden showed fewer deaths from breast cancer in women who took estrogens.

HRT and Breast Cancer Survivors

If you're a breast cancer survivor, will ERT make you more susceptible to a recurrence? Surprisingly, no study has yet shown an increased risk for such women. A recent Australian study reports that 90 breast cancer survivors who took estrogen actually had a lower disease recurrence rate than breast cancer survivors who didn't take estrogens. Hence, the suggestion is that estrogens may protect from further disease episodes. The study's short-coming, however, was that it followed these women for only two to three years. Moreover, participants were not randomly selected. A greater number of longer-term randomized studies are needed to address this question adequately.

The Effects of Progestins and Androgens on Breast Cancer

Older research yielded conflicting data in regard to progestins' effects on breast tissue when added to estrogen therapy. However, recent data—although limited—suggest that added progestins appear to neither significantly increase nor decrease the risk for breast cancer. Since most studies to date have evaluated the effects of only ERT on breast cancer, the added effects of progestins await closer scrutiny.

In a 1994 issue of the journal *Menopause,* Drs. John C. Arpels and Robert D. Nachtigall went so far as to suggest that the absence of naturally circulating progesterone in the postmenopausal body may open the door to a greater risk for malignancies such as breast cancer later in life. After menopause, there is no progesterone to counterbalance the activity of the remaining amounts of naturally produced estrogen. The authors theorize that this could pose a greater threat of estrogen-induced cellular over-

---

"I thought that maybe progestin supplements like Provera would counteract any risk of breast cancer—since they do that for endometrial cancer. But there's no sign they do, according to my doctor."

growth. New data from the Nurses' Health Study, however, suggest that progestins don't protect breast tissue from estrogenic effects, nor do they add to it.

While more research is needed to know more about how replacement androgens affect breast tissue, they are not thought to increase the risk for cancer. A few studies show that when androgens are given to women who have a history of breast cancer, their cancer regressed. Androgen therapy has also been associated with an improved survival rate in metastatic breast cancer patients. The fact that breast cancer is much less prevalent among men than women has prompted speculation that a man's higher levels of androgen might help reduce this cancer. No doubt many other factors play into a woman's greater susceptibility.

As you can see, weighing the benefits and risks of hormone replacement therapy can be complicated. I urge you to work actively with your doctor to see how your health profile affects this deeply personal decision.

If you decide that HRT is right for you, your next decision is to select among the many available preparations and regimens. The next chapter will help you make that informed choice.

7

Hormone Replacement: A Growing Number of Options

If you've decided that hormone replacement is right for you, you'll quickly discover that there are so many different types of hormones, approved dosages, routes of administration, and possible medication schedules, that you'll be tempted to leave the medical details to your doctor. To illustrate just how many replacement options are available, a survey team discovered that 283 Los Angeles physicians were prescribing 84 different hormone replacement regimens for their patients. And the options continue to grow!

Your physician is there to recommend the HRT package that best suits you. That said, I urge you to be an active participant in this decision by becoming aware of the pros and cons of different medication timetables, the convenience or inconvenience associated with the various ways of taking medication, and the promising products that someday could make hormone therapy more effective and easier to manage.

"It's important for women to ask questions about various regimens and open up a dialogue with their physicians," notes Irma L. Mebane-Sims, NIH epidemiologist and program administrator for the PEPI trial. "Women are apt to think that different replacement schedules are based on rigorous scientific experiments, but they aren't. Initially the prescribing habits for replacement therapy simply mimicked the different ways oral contraceptives were administered. We fell into them." In other words, available regimens aren't set in stone, and one approach isn't necessarily better than another. All the more reason to hunt out a regimen that suits your particular needs.

In the past decade the number of new hormone products and treatment techniques has mushroomed—a trend likely to continue as the first of the baby boomers turn 50 in 1996. (According to the U.S. Census Bureau, the number of women aged 45 to 54 is projected to grow by 73 percent during this decade and the next.) If you begin HRT, many physicians will recommend the regimens and products that have been used most widely, because their associated risks, benefits, and side effects have been the most thoroughly studied.

Different Hormone Preparations: Which One's Right for You?

When settling on a hormone replacement approach, you and your doctor first need to decide how the medication will be delivered to your body. *Oral* preparations—tablets taken by mouth—reach the bloodstream by way of the gastrointestinal tract and a "first pass" through the liver. Estrogens, progestins, and androgens can all be taken orally. *Nonoral* preparations, in comparison, aren't swallowed or ingested, and therefore avoid the intestines and subsequent major passage through the liver. As you'll see, whether or not a preparation follows the intestinal tract can sometimes make a difference in how it affects you.

Available nonoral routes for estrogens include transdermal (literally, through the skin) patches, injections, and vaginal creams. Nonoral estrogen forms available in other countries, but not yet marketed in the United States, include *subcutaneous* (under the skin) pellets, vaginal rings, and estrogen gel. Available nonoral progestins consist of injections and vaginal suppositories. Although either not approved for HRT use or not yet available on the U.S. market, HRT transdermal progestins, HRT progesterone intrauterine devices, and an HRT vaginal progesterone gel are in the development and/or review stages.

You may choose just one route of administration—taking all your hormones in tablet form, for instance. Oral tablets are the most common formulation for hormone therapy. Or you might use a combination of routes. If your uterus is intact, your physician might prescribe, for example, estrogens delivered nonorally through a skin patch in conjunction with orally administered progestin tablets.

Supplemental estrogens can cause side effects in 5 to 10 percent of women, with most reported as being only mildly disruptive. You may experience nausea, bloating, breast tenderness, and headaches as well as spot bleeding or a return of menstrual bleeding. More women experience side effects from progestins; over 50 percent of users are apt to feel progestin's PMS-like symptoms to some degree, especially at the onset of treatment when your dosage usually requires a period of adjustment. The higher the progestin dose, the greater your chance of experiencing water retention, bloating, breast tenderness, irritability, mood swings and anxiety, constipation, and irregular uterine bleeding. The withdrawal bleeding that often follows each cycle of progestin use is the most frequent reason for women going off progestins. If you were prone to PMS in your premenopausal years, you may be susceptible to progestin's PMS-like aspects.

By some reports, changing the route of administration—say from ingested pill to skin patch or to injection—can help relieve HRT's side effects for some women.

Let's review the different hormone preparations and their advantages and disadvantages.

Oral Estrogen Tablets

Oral estrogen preparations need to be taken daily, save for one oral type—quinestrol (brand name: Estrovis)—which you take once a week.

ADVANTAGES
One advantage that oral tablets have over other routes is that they are the most studied and time-proven route of replacement therapy, especially with respect to one type of estrogen, conjugated equine estrogens (CEE). There are less thorough data to tell us how hormones administered nonorally affect various systems. As these alternative pathways are scrutinized, however, the more their suspected benefits are being validated.

A second possible advantage is that when oral estrogens, unlike those administered nonorally, make a "first pass" through the liver, their effect on the liver's regulation of cholesterol has been associated with a marked increase in HDL, the "good" cholesterol. It's uncertain if nonoral estrogens—which don't undergo a direct pass through the liver—can raise HDL so appreciably, although there's evidence that supplemental estrogens administered either orally or nonorally may provide heart protection through a complex network of changes. Estrogens' effects on HDL might be only part of the story.

Disadvantages

When you take hormones by mouth, their passage through the metabolically active intestines and liver can sometimes create complications. Therefore, if you have a liver disorder, your doctor may advise against estrogens as well as androgens and synthetic progestins. Also, as hormones pass through your stomach, you may feel nauseated. Another possible disadvantage is that when tablets are swallowed, their absorption rate through the intestinal wall may be variable, leading to inadequate hormone levels in the bloodstream. On the other hand, the skin can also be responsible for variable absorption rates when the patch is used.

Micronized (Oral) Estrogens

Micronized estrogens are different from other oral estrogens in that they consist of much smaller particles of estrogens (estradiol). The original theory behind them was that, because they were already fragmented, they'd break down less than other replacement estrogens when crossing the liver, and as a result retain more of their estradiol structure. This would give users more circulating estradiol, the female body's primary estrogen. This theory hasn't been validated. We now know that, postmenopausally, most oral estradiol gets converted in a woman's body to estrone, a less active estrogen. Therefore micronized estradiol is converted predominantly to estrone, not predominantly to estradiol. This product isn't by any means inferior; as long as they are taken in adequate doses, all approved replacement estrogens deliver comparable estrogenic effects.

Some claim that estradiol products are more "natural" than conjugated equine estrogens (CEE), since the former are primarily derived from the ovarian-made estrogen most in evidence before menopause, as opposed to the hormones derived from horses that primarily make up CEE. However, no studies have yet indicated that estradiol-based estrogens are a better or worse replacement measure than conjugated equine estrogens (which contain some estradiol).

In the United States, micronized estradiol is available as the brand name Estrace. While micronization does not necessarily make this preparation more effective than other available estrogens, it appears to be in every way equal.

MEDICATION TIPS

• Six different types of generic oral estrogens are available, all of which have been proven effective for menopausal use: conjugated equine estrogens, esterified estrogens, micronized estradiol, estropipate, ethinyl estradiol, and quinestrol. No one type has been demonstrated to be more effective than the others.

• Each type of estrogen can be prepared in different doses. Bear in mind that each estrogen has its own particular potency, which explains why the dosages vary from one to another. Your doctor will prescribe the dosage that carries the least amount of risk associated with your particular health needs. Examples of typical dose ranges used for menopausal symptoms include: 0.3 to 1.25 mg for conjugated equine estrogens; 0.625 to 1.25 mg for estropipate; 0.5 to 2.0 mg for micronized estradiol.

Oral Progestin Tablets

Generally, replacement therapy uses oral progestins synthesized in the laboratory instead of progesterone, the natural form of the ovarian hormone. Physicians prescribe oral progesterone far less because it breaks down in the liver and can produce metabolites with sedativelike side effects. However, a modified oral progesterone tablet developed by Schering-Plough is currently under review in this country. If such a product could overcome the metabolic obstacles, it might carry certain advantages; for example, it might not block the estrogen-associated rise in good cholesterol (HDL), as some synthetic progestins have been observed to do.

All oral progestins marketed in this country are prepared for daily use. As will be discussed later in this chapter, some regimens call for use of progestins every day; others are based on a monthly start-and-stop schedule of progestins.

ADVANTAGES
The effects of progestins taken orally are better researched and understood than those associated with nonoral progestins. When combined with replacement estrogens, 10 mg of oral medroxyprogesterone acetate, or an equivalent progestin, is known to cancel out the estrogen-provoked risk of endometrial overgrowth.

DISADVANTAGES
Oral progestins may be inadvisable for women with liver disorders. Moreover, there is some evidence that certain oral synthetic progestins, when taken with estrogens, reduce estrogens' HDL-cholesterol benefits. Findings from

the PEPI trial suggest that if, instead, oral micronized progesterone is taken with estrogens, the cholesterol benefits remain nearly as substantial as when estrogens are taken alone.

MICRONIZED (ORAL) PROGESTERONE

When progesterone is micronized (ground down into minute particles) and taken orally, it is more easily absorbed and can more effectively cross the liver than regularly prepared progesterone. Some women tolerate it better than synthetic progestins. Data from the PEPI trial indicate that its use in conjunction with estrogens allows for an HDL-cholesterol increase that is substantially higher than when medroxyprogesterone acetate (MPA) is added to estrogen. (Currently, MPA is the most widely sold progestin.) Yet micronized progesterone is just as protective of the endometrium as MPA.

Nonoral: Transdermal Patch

For many women, the estrogen transdermal patch, which began commercial sales in this country in 1986, can be as efficient as a tablet in delivering estrogens into the bloodstream and in treating menopausal symptoms such as hot flashes and vaginal dryness. The patch has been shown to prevent bone loss. However, whether or not it can protect a woman against heart disease to the extent that estrogens do hasn't been fully assessed. However, there's every reason to believe that the patch will prove to be as effective as the tablet.

ADVANTAGES

Changed once or twice a week (depending upon the brand used) and usually worn on the abdomen or buttocks, this self-adhering skin patch steadily releases estradiol through a semipermeable membrane into the skin and blood vessels, quickly sending estrogens into general circulation. This constant release of medication is more sustained, hence preferable, some researchers believe, to oral estrogens' initial surge into the bloodstream.

Moreover, since hormones from the patch initially circumvent the stomach and liver, some women with liver disorders can use them. And because transdermal hormones travel more directly to the cells than orally introduced hormones, less medication gets "lost" in the process. Hence, the doses used for transdermal hormones and other nonoral routes can be lower than oral doses while achieving the same biological effects. For example, while the low-dose patch delivers 0.05 mg/day of estradiol, the lowest daily oral dose of the same estradiol is 0.5 mg/day—ten times the transdermal amount. When oral estradiol crosses the liver, it becomes estrone, the much less potent estrogen. Manufacturers put higher doses of estrogens into oral tablets knowing that their potency will diminish by the time they reach the cells.

> "After I started wearing the estrogen patch, my daytime hot flashes disappeared almost immediately. My night sweats took longer to go away, but they were mostly gone in a week to ten days."

Since the patch delivers lower amounts of estrogen than oral tablets do, there's speculation that the patch's lower dose of estrogens could prove a safer route for women with a family or personal history of estrogen-related cancers. However, this theory is far from proven.

Unlike oral estradiol, the patch's estradiol doesn't get converted to estrone. A woman using it ends up with estradiol circulating in the blood—the primary premenopausal estrogen that menopause has depleted. Estradiol's effects in the postmenopausal body haven't been proven better or worse than other estrogens. But some women like the idea that they're putting premenopausal estrogens back into circulation.

Probably the patch's most alluring feature is that its once- or twice-a-week schedule is simpler to deal with than daily pill-taking. This convenience is somewhat reduced for women with intact uteruses who may also need to take oral progestins for endometrial protection, since no progestin patches are yet marketed. Until recently the only estrogen patch available in this country has been Estraderm (CIBA) which provides a four-day supply of estrogens. Your doctor will advise changing it every $3^{1}/_{2}$ days, or twice a week, to ensure that the patch's contents don't run low and that a steady rate of estrogens enters the bloodstream.

Several seven-day estrogen transdermal systems offered by different makers are coming to market, upping the convenience factor. Climara (Berlex), for instance, provides 0.05 mg of estradiol a day through a newly developed adhesive matrix backing.

CIBA has introduced a new patch that contains four doses—0.375, 0.05, 0.75, and 1.0 mg of estradiol. These patches need to be changed twice a week.

DISADVANTAGES

Despite all there is to recommend it, the patch has some drawbacks. Some women don't absorb transdermally delivered medications as successfully as others. Also, 10 percent of women who use the patch find that it irritates their skin. New matrix backing, as opposed to the older patch's use of a liquid reservoir for release of medication, should produce less irritation.

More significantly, because nonoral routes represent a newer form of administration than oral HRT, less is known about their long-term influence on bone loss and heart disease. The FDA has approved the patch for treatment of menopausal symptoms, with solid evidence showing that transdermal estrogens relieve hot flashes and vaginal dryness. The patch also has been approved for the prevention of osteoporosis, with studies giving clear signs that transdermal estrogens retard bone loss. Transdermal estrogens appear to be as effective as oral estrogens in inhibiting the accelerated period of bone loss seen after menopause. But they haven't been used long enough for researchers to be able to judge their long-term effects on bone fracture.

The patch's outcome on heart disease also requires more analysis. One study suggests that some oral estrogens (CEEs), in fact, may function more as antioxidants—factors that help the body guard against disease. This could mean that CEEs are more effective than the patch at thwarting atherosclerosis. Currently, there's indication that longer durations of transdermal estrogens bestow at least a small yet significant rise in HDL. However, in terms of a positive effect on HDL/LDL, studies show that the patch may not be as effective as oral estrogens. Nonetheless, there are signs that both transdermal and oral estrogens impact the cardiovascular system in numerous other ways—not just at the level of the lipids. But whether or not the patch's overall effects match those achieved with oral estrogens still needs proof.

In other words, transdermal hormones provide the same biological benefits that orally administered hormones do, but to what extent remains unclear. Until fuller analysis can provide more evidence that, long-term, the patch protects bone and heart as effectively as oral estrogens do, the latter will probably remain the standard. At this point the research indicates that transdermal systems yield the same benefits provided by their oral counterparts.

FUTURE PROSPECTS

A skin patch that combines both estrogens and progestins is available throughout the United Kingdom and in several European countries. It contains less than one-quarter of the progestins that oral progestins contain, since less medication is generally needed when the gastrointestinal tract is bypassed. Because of its lower doses, women experience fewer progestin-related side effects, according to CIBA, its maker. A similar system is being developed in this country, but it could take years of testing before its combination of drugs is FDA-approved. A patch solely for the administration of progestins is also under development.

> "I find the most comfortable place to wear the patch is on the abdomen, below the navel. Each time you put one on, you need to change its location slightly; putting it on the same spot possibly irritates the skin. I have friends who wear it on the buttocks, but for me it was itchy there."

MEDICATION TIPS

• The estrogen patch is prepared in two doses: 0.05 mg/day and 0.1 mg/day. Physicians are likely to begin by prescribing the lower dose. However, because of varying absorption rates through the skin, some women need the higher dose to relieve menopausal symptoms. If symptoms continue, an easily administered blood test can measure how much of the patch's estradiol is actually reaching the bloodstream. (It's thought that a level of estradiol greater than 100 pg/ml relieves most hot flashes.) No such simple clinical test exists for orally-administered conjugated equine estrogens. CEEs contain different compounds that make them impractical to measure.

• To date, the once-a-week patches that are coming on the market also are prepared in two doses: 0.05 mg/day and 0.1 mg/day.

• Just like oral estrogens, estrogens administered transdermally will make their way to uterine cells via the bloodstream. Hence, for a woman with an intact uterus who is using the patch, the use of progestins is recommended for endometrial protection.

> "I use two patches at once because my absorption rate is low. My family always knows when I need to change to new patches—I get irritable when low on hormones."

Intravenous and Intramuscular Hormone Injections

Estrogens and androgens can also be injected *intravenously* (into veins) or *intramuscularly* (into muscles). Intramuscular injections are usually the preferred route, with intravenous therapy often reserved for emergency situations that warrant faster acting therapy, as in cases of irregular bleeding that is so heavy it needs to be stopped immediately. When androgens are injected, doctors regularly combine them with injected estrogens.

Progestin injectables aren't typically used for hormone replacement. When they are, progesterone is apt to be injected intramuscularly in an oil solution, which helps to dissolve the hormone before it reaches the bloodstream. More commonly, injected progesterone is used as a contraceptive. Depo-Provera, one such product, received FDA approval in 1992.

The long-term effects of injected hormones have not been thoroughly determined.

ADVANTAGES

Not a common HRT administration method, injectables are used by less than 1 percent of women. Yet in certain parts of the country, and among certain groups of doctors, this route is very popular, particularly because one injection can allow high levels of hormones to circulate over long periods of time. (Only implanted pellets, if approved by the FDA, would offer a longer duration of hormone therapy.) When women experience severe hot flashes after the removal of both ovaries, the potency of this delivery form has been observed to alleviate flashes more effectively than other routes. Injected hormones are also apt to be used immediately after surgical menopause because they bypass the stomach and its postoperative sensitivity to food or oral medication.

For the sake of convenience, women whose daytime activities make it hard to get to the doctor's office for an injection can learn how to inject themselves at home.

> "I have six children and life is pretty hectic. That's why I learned how to inject progesterone into my hip. It saves going into the doctor's office once a month and has worked out beautifully. There's only once hitch: The needle is very long, so, psychologically, it takes getting used to. But it's a very fine, thin needle, so it doesn't hurt at all."

DISADVANTAGES

When a hormone preparation is injected, its levels tend to be higher during the first few weeks of the treatment period and lower the last few weeks. Other routes that dispense hormones more evenly over time are thought to provide more reliable treatment. Once a dose is injected, it stays in the system until all of it is metabolized, which can take many months. This can be problematic if unforeseen side effects occur, since there is no way to stop or reduce the dosage once the hormone is in the bloodstream. Clinical observations by some researchers have found that the potency of this route can sometimes foster a dependency on estrogens.

MEDICATION TIPS

• One injected dose can deliver up to a three-month supply of hormones.

• Similar to oral estrogens, injected estrogens also can pose an increased cancer risk to the endometrium. Therefore, a woman with an intact uterus who is receiving estrogen injections will mostly likely need progestins as well. Progestins taken for one week for each month that injected estrogens are circulating in a woman's blood system can protect the uterus from hyperplasia.

• Products that combine estrogens and androgens

(testosterone) in one injection conveniently dispense both hormones simultaneously.

Vaginal Estrogen Creams

Estrogen creams applied vaginally are absorbed by cellular tissue and make their way into underlying blood vessels. Research has found that postmenopausal women initially absorb vaginal preparations more readily than pre-menopausal women. This is probably because vaginal tissue after menopause becomes thinner, and replacement estrogens pass through the skin and into the blood more readily. As treated tissues recover, absorption rates are apt to lessen since estrogens won't travel through the estrogen-thickened tissue as quickly. Vaginal doses might be reduced at this point, yet they will need to be continued indefinitely in order to maintain the vaginal tissue's health.

ADVANTAGES

Because they build up postmenopausal vaginal tissue, vaginal estrogen creams can efficiently treat vaginal dryness, *dyspareunia* (painful intercourse), and other urogenital symptoms brought on by the depletion of natural hormones. The estrogen amounts employed vaginally are often smaller than nonvaginal doses used for treating hot flashes or bone loss. While some reports indicate that estrogen creams can subdue hot flashes, this remains questionable, especially given the variable absorption rate of vaginal creams. Even though some applications of these creams are equivalent to doses above 0.3 oral CEEs, since women use them less often (three times a week or less), they get less total medication weekly. The fact that not all the cream applied gets absorbed further reduces the overall dosage.

In some cases, you can use vaginal estrogens if oral estrogens are ruled out because of a liver disorder. If your gynecologist prescribes vaginal estrogens, make sure to inform your family physician; your liver should be periodically monitored for any adverse effects if there is a history of liver disorder.

If you've previously had breast cancer, many doctors might withhold these creams. Yet there's no hard evidence that breast cancer survivors who use these preparations are at a higher risk for a cancer recurrence. Sometimes physicians will suggest this route for estrogens after first consulting with a patient's oncologist.

It's unclear what dosage of vaginal estrogens can effectively treat urinary tract infections. But some clues may be taken from the Israel-based study mentioned in the last chapter. The women who participated in that study benefited from an estrogen vaginal cream (one roughly equivalent to standard vaginal cream doses found in the United States) that was used nightly for two weeks followed by twice-weekly applications for eight months. The study underscores the value of aggressively treating women with a history of urinary tract infections with estrogen cream during the first few weeks, then tapering treatment.

DISADVANTAGES

Vaginal estrogens are intended to work locally on the areas where cream is applied. Yet it's now known that these preparations can be absorbed into the bloodstream and circulate systemically, or throughout the body. It's uncertain how much estrogen travels beyond the vagina, but especially in the case of smaller doses, it's not considered to be enough to protect against heart disease. In the case of larger doses, however, it may be enough to cause unwanted reactions. If you have a liver ailment, your liver ought to be tested after beginning vaginal estrogens to ensure that estrogens aren't unduly stressing that organ.

The observation that vaginal estrogen creams can enter the blood suggests that they may also benefit bone and other estrogen-receptive locations. However, when bone loss is a problem, vaginal estrogen creams do not provide strong enough treatment. These creams aren't prescribed in high enough doses over a sustained period of time to meet that need.

Vaginal creams can be messy to use. Once you apply a cream by applicator into your vagina or spread it over urogenital tissue by finger, it can become more liquidy and leak. Applying a cream just before bedtime can reduce vaginal leakage, thereby improving absorption. Note that these creams are not meant to be used as a lubricant for intercourse and don't work in that capacity.

MEDICATION TIPS

• Applying an estrogen cream three times a week can usually improve vaginal dryness in two to eight weeks. A recent study showed that the low dose of 0.3 mg of conjugated estrogen cream can be effective. If your vaginal tissues show no improvement, your doctor may recommend that you increase applications to four times a week. When your tissues start responding, you can lower applications to twice a week, or even less as long as your symptoms are minimized.

• No matter what dosage of estrogen cream is used vaginally, some of it almost always is absorbed into the bloodstream. This means that with even small doses, you and your physician should be aware that the cream might stimulate some growth of the lining of the uterus, and that you may need progestins in addition to estrogen cream.

• If your uterus is intact and you start using vaginal estrogen creams three times weekly, I recommend you add progestins for a week at a time, four times a year, to protect the endometrium. An easy-to-remember timetable is to start progestins at the beginning of each new season: spring, summer, winter, and fall.

• Several different preparations of vaginal estrogen creams are marketed and all are equally effective. The different types of estrogens they contain include dienestrol, estropipate, estradiol, and conjugated equine estrogens.

• Vaginal estrogen creams may provide you with more complete treatment for vaginal dryness and other vaginal symptoms than do oral or transdermal estrogens. Although a woman taking an oral dose of 0.625 CEE for hot flashes, heart protection, or bone maintenance may also get the side benefit of improved vaginal tissues, it's not a sure thing. (Note: Exogenous estrogens are not approved by the FDA for heart protection.)

Progesterone Suppositories

As mentioned, when progestins are needed to counter the risk of estrogen-stimulated endometrial growth, physicians don't normally prescribe oral progesterone because it breaks down in the body and has sedativelike effects.

Progesterone introduced nonorally and vaginally largely avoids these problems. While not considered standard treatment, physicians may prescribe vaginal progesterone suppositories, especially in cases in which a woman doesn't tolerate the PMS-like side effects caused by synthetic oral progestins. Progesterone suppositories may possibly produce fewer side effects, because their doses are less potent than oral doses. Nonetheless, they may still have some PMS-like repercussions. Because medication can leak out of the vagina, suppositories can be messy, and for this reason some women may not care for them.

More frequently, progesterone suppositories are used to treat infertility. In this role, they help to prepare an endometrium that can sustain pregnancy.

What's the Future for HRT?

Subcutaneous Estrogen Implants

Although estrogen-containing pellets aren't yet commercially available in this country, they are reportedly very popular in Britain, Australia, and South Africa and are gaining attention in France and Scandinavia as an effective and affordable hormone replacement route. "Because pill-taking and even patches are hard to comply with, my educated guess is that when the research gets done and passed by the FDA, these implants may prove a superior route," said Dr. Donald P. Swartz, head of the Division of General Gynecology at Albany Medical College.

Implanted in fatty tissue beneath the skin, these biodegradable pellets, each the size of a corn kernel, release estrogens at a slow, constant rate into the circulatory system for up to six consecutive months. What's immediately obvious about this form of administration is that for months at a time it does away with the "nuisance factor" of complying to a drug-taking schedule.

There are promising signs that this newly advanced HRT route reduces bone loss and protects against heart disease, but to what degree remains under study. The insertion of the pellet requires a minor surgical procedure. Should therapy need to be halted because of an unforeseen health condition or other reason, the implant can be difficult to remove, one of the downsides that has reportedly stalled FDA approval.

Vaginal Estrogen Rings

Available outside the United States—though currently being developed and tested here—vaginal estrogen rings someday may provide women in this country with a convenient way of relieving vaginal dryness. If they dispense high enough doses of estrogens, these rings could possibly also protect the bones and the heart. Inserted into the vagina and fitted around the cervix, they carry the advantage of dispensing a predictable, sustained release of estrogens for up to three months per ring.

A large majority of women tested noted no discomfort from the ring. Although its developers claim this device can be left in place during intercourse, sexual activity can dislodge it. However, like a diaphragm, the vaginal ring can be easily inserted or removed—for intercourse or to halt side effects. Also, it can reduce the leakage problem encountered with vaginal creams. A possible disadvantage is that this device may be uncomfortable for an older woman whose vagina has decreased in size. It may also prove difficult to use for a woman who has had a hysterectomy and has no cervix to anchor it to.

Intrauterine Progesterone Device

The progesterone intrauterine devices currently on the market are used solely for contraceptive purposes. However, researchers in this country have begun looking into the feasibility of employing such devices for hormone therapy. The early outlook is promising. In one study, albeit a small one, women using a progesterone IUD placed in the uterus along with daily oral estrogens experienced no withdrawal bleeding and no PMS-like side effects. If larger studies bear out such advantages, there may soon be the option of an IUD that could effectively release progesterone over the course of six to twelve months. This device would most likely have the usual drawbacks of an IUD, such as possible infection, uterine puncture, and loss of the device out of the uterus.

Estrogen Skin Gel

Reported to be the leading hormone replacement product used in France, an estrogen gel is currently under review in this country. Rubbed on the abdomen or thighs, this product is said to act on menopausal symptoms and systemic conditions the same way the transdermal patch does—by dispatching medication to blood vessels directly beneath the skin. It therefore may provide bone and heart protection equivalent to what investigators are finding the patch provides. Possible problems with this product include the large area of skin that needs to covered for effective results, a variable absorption rate, and difficulty with dosage control.

Vaginal Progesterone Gel

According to its developers (Columbia Laboratories), a newly developed vaginal progesterone gel administered in small doses has the ability to fully guard the endometrium against estrogen-provoked overgrowth. Not yet marketed, the gel and its feasibility as a treatment form are currently being reviewed by the FDA.

Applied by applicator into the vagina, each 45-mg dose of progesterone is targeted specifically for uterine cells and is sustained-released over a two-day period. The gel's nonoral route may mean it won't reduce estrogen-boosted HDL levels the way oral synthetic progestins have been observed to do.

Since this gel would directly treat the vagina and probably the uterus, the doses administered vaginally would be less than those administered orally. The dose associated with this gel contains one-seventh of the progestational hormone found in an oral dose. Therefore, it could possibly help reduce the PMS-like side effects that higher doses of oral progestins provoke.

Types of Exogenous Hormones: Is Natural Or Synthetic Better?

The chemical basis for replacement estrogens and progestins varies from product to product. For instance, micronized estradiol goes into Estrace (Mead Johnson), esterified estrogens make up Estratab (Solvay), and ethinyl estradiol is the basis for Estinyl (Schering). How do you choose among all these varying compounds? Are some better than others?

By and large, replacement estrogens, no matter their chemical makeup, have the same biological effects depending on the route by which they are administered. The estrogens most frequently prescribed in this country are conjugated equine estrogens (CEE). Composed of as many as ten different types of estrogen, including the human estrogens estrone and estradiol, CEEs are primarily based

on estrogens extracted from the urine of pregnant mares—
hence the brand name Premarin. (Like humans, horses
produce more sex hormones when they're pregnant.)
Judging from the effects of conjugated equine estrogens,
they achieve the same results in the female body as human
hormones do, although differences in efficacy have not
been thoroughly tested.

Instead of conjugated equine estrogens, some estrogen
products are based on estrone, the estrogen most prominent in postmenopausal women. In others, the primary
agent is estradiol, the estrogen most in evidence before
menopause. Again, there doesn't appear to be any major
difference in the efficacy of these two chemical bases. Even
though estrone is a less potent estrogen than estradiol, its
potency level is compensated for through dosage.

Certain makers of replacement estrogens tout their
product as being "natural" as opposed to synthetic, since
the hormone ingredients are pure forms of what the
human body makes, or, in the case of Premarin, what the
horse makes. Some people are apt to think "natural" is
better than "synthetic," but this isn't necessarily so. All
"synthetic" means is that during the laboratory process a
hormone's base compounds have been altered, usually
only for the sake of making it metabolically more efficient.

Lab alterations can improve a hormone's absorption,
help it weather the turbulence of metabolism, or increase
its potency. Many of the confusing chemical names of supplemental hormones simply refer to the type of lab processing a particular hormone has undergone. Take
piperazine estrone sulfate, for instance. "Piperazine"
refers to the attachment of a molecule to the estrone compound that helps protect it from metabolic breakdown. In
ethinyl estradiol, "ethinyl" indicates the addition of an

ethinyl compound that prevents too much estradiol from being broken down in the liver so more of it will be absorbed into the blood.

As already noted, most supplemental progestins are synthesized in order to offer the patient a more effective hormone than what oral progesterone provides. When taken orally, pure progesterone breaks apart rapidly in the liver and gets excreted, so ineffectual amounts get absorbed into the bloodstream. It can also produce metabolites that can cause drowsiness. Slightly altering progesterone's molecular structure in the laboratory greatly reduces these problems. Some alterations result in synthetic progestins that bear similarities to androgens. Other alterations lead to less androgenic compounds— medroxyprogesterone acetate (MPA), for instance, the most widely used progestin in this country. Akin to the complicated-sounding names given to estrogens, the names of progestins and androgens often reflect what type of laboratory process has transpired. "Medroxy acetate," for instance, indicates the change in progesterone's structure to make it more chemically stable when crossing the liver.

Whether "natural" or "synthetic," very often the final product has gone through some refinement in the lab. In the case of conjugated equine estrogens, which are sometimes referred to as "natural," estrogens have been rendered more water soluble for the sake of absorption. In the case of micronized estradiol, estrogens have been broken down to assist their absorption. All in all, you shouldn't let the terms "natural" or "synthetic" sway you one way or the other in regard to an HRT product. Such terms say little about the product's underlying integrity.

In the making of all estrogens, as well as progestins and

androgens, the goal is to ensure that the drug that enters the body ends up circulating at levels that contribute to the desired effects. The aim of standard doses of estrogens is to put estrogens back into the body that are comparable to premenopausal levels seen early in the menstrual cycle's follicular phase. These levels on average are lower than those seen later in the cycle.

Most replacement preparations are available in more than one dose. Oral Premarin, for instance, is prepared in five different dosages: 0.3 mg, 0.625 mg, 0.9 mg, 1.25 mg, and 2.5 mg, the highest. Doses are prescribed according to the intensity of the symptom or condition being treated, as well as a woman's health status and ability to tolerate a certain dose. A general rule of thumb with prescribed estrogens is to start with a middle-of-the-road dose, weigh its effects, then alter dosage if need be.

What's the Best Schedule for You?

When you embark on hormone replacement therapy, you're going to discover that along with a variety of hormone types, dosages, and administration routes, a wide selection of timetables exist, especially when you're taking a combination of hormones. You may start out on one schedule, become dissatisfied with it, and try another. Fitting the right dose and hormone type with the right administration route with the right schedule can take adjustments and time, not to mention patience on your part. An ideal regimen is one that would offer a no-hassle medication schedule without side effects. Although it's unreasonable to think there will ever be one perfect HRT approach that fits all women, HRT products and regimens are constantly being modified to make them easier to use.

Only you can determine which is most manageable and convenient for you.

Combined Estrogen-Progestin Therapy

If you have an intact uterus and require endometrial-protecting progestins along with estrogens, the two most commonly employed medication schedules are *sequential combined therapy* and *continuous combined therapy*. To date, there's no evidence that one is safer or more effective than the other. Both carry advantages and disadvantages that may be a deciding factor for you.

The most widely used HRT medication schedule—sequential combined therapy—attempts to mimic a woman's natural, premenopausal ovarian hormone cycle. Although many different sequential approaches have come into use, when following the standard timetable you take supplemental estrogens for days 1 through 25 each month, and add on progestins anywhere from day 13 to 16 and lasting through day 25. These staggered levels of hormones result in menstrual-like withdrawal bleeding in a reported 92 percent of women using this approach. This bleeding occurs because replacement estrogens and progestins alter the growth of the endometrium; when progestins are withdrawn, bleeding occurs. (Note how this mimics a woman's natural menstrual cycle: As progesterone levels fall toward the end of the cycle, bleeding occurs.) Withdrawal bleeding almost always follows a term of progestin use and is generally less heavy than regular menstrual bleeding and accompanied by fewer cramps. This artificial period normally starts on day 21 or later. Sometimes withdrawal bleeding doesn't occur, which need not be a concern. However, if any bleeding occurs other than when expected, you need to report it to your doctor, since it could signal an abnormal situation.

The obvious drawback with combined sequential therapy is that it carries the inconvenience of a period, just at an age when you might have been looking forward to life without tampons, pads, and messiness. Nonetheless, many physicians recommend this approach because it's been used longer and more extensively than other schedules, and has the advantage of being time-tested.

> "I began sequential therapy, but became annoyed with the cramping and monthly bleeding, so I stopped and tried continuous therapy. Well, the bleeding with that schedule bothered me too, so I tried sequential again. Believe it or not, once more the periods got to me and I returned to continuous therapy, this time determined to stick it out. In three to four months no bleeding was occurring."

An increasingly popular alternative, continuous combined therapy, calls for both estrogens and progestins to be taken every day of the month, 365 days a year. This usually results in a complete absence of bleeding within three to six months of the therapy's onset. The concept behind this approach is that the continuous use of estrogens and progestins exhausts hormone receptors in the uterus to the point where the uterine lining stops growing and therefore stops being sloughed off to result in menstruation.

Limited data indicate that most of those who remain on this schedule do stop bleeding within a year. The problem with this approach is that few women are willing to tolerate the irregular bleeding in the beginning months. In fact, up to 50 percent of women reportedly abandon continu-

Figure 8. Estrogen-Progestin Regimens

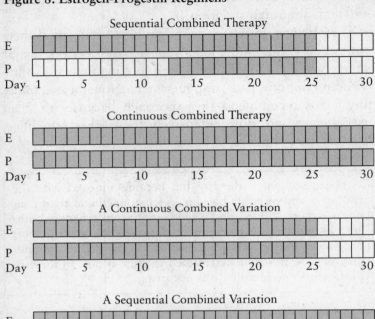

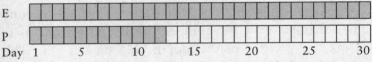

Sequential combined therapy *and* continuous combined therapy *represent the two most commonly employed estrogen-progestin medication schedules. However, in attempts to maintain endometrial protection as well as minimize side effects, many regimen variations are also in use.*

Source: *Menopause Management,* November/December 1993.

ous combined therapy within the first six months of treatment. This regimen has been observed to work better with older women; they're apt to experience less bleeding, probably because their uterine lining is less responsive to hormones.

When breakthrough bleeding occurs, a physician cannot immediately determine if the bleeding is caused by supplemental hormones or is related to hyperplasia or some other condition. Hence, every bleeding episode may require evaluation. The technique of transvaginal ultrasound (see Chapter 6, p. 167) makes it easier to measure for endometrial overgrowth. Some cases may require an endometrial biopsy, often an uncomfortable procedure. If irregular bleeding keeps recurring, frequent endometrial evaluations of any kind can turn this therapy into more of a chore than a benefit.

> "When I started continuous estrogen-progestin therapy, the worst part was that I didn't know when I was going to bleed. It got to be really irritating, so I changed to a sequential pattern. At least now I know when I'll bleed."

Along with the prospect of loss of bleeding, what recruits some women to this schedule, however, are progestin doses that are lower than those used in sequential therapy and thus freer of PMS-like side effects. Continuous therapy doses can be lower (e.g. 2.5 mg/day/MPA) because progestin use is stretched out over the entire month

> Martha Marean, an MGH gynecologic nurse/clinician, recounts: "One patient who was ten years older than her husband opted for sequential therapy over continuous because she liked the idea that with sequential therapy she'd keep having monthly bleeding. She wanted her husband to perceive her as a woman whose menstrual cycles hadn't stopped. If she'd chosen continuous therapy, she'd have no monthly bleeding."

rather than taken in a concentrated ten- to thirteen-days-per-month stretch, as in sequential therapy.

Since continuous therapy is a newer regimen than sequential therapy, its long-term effects on postmenopausal women are less well researched. It's thought to provide the same long-term benefits for heart and bone, however.

Physicians and researchers are continuing to hunt for a combined estrogen-progestin schedule that's both convenient and relatively free of side effects. Consequently, standard sequential and continuous regimens have given rise to numerous hybrids. To give a few examples:

• Estrogens (pills or patch) are used continuously, with progestins sequentially added during days 1 to 12. Normal withdrawal bleeding in this case occurs after day 10. Some women like this timetable because it's easier for them to remember to take progestins at the beginning of the month.

• Estrogens are used continuously, with progestins added for ten to fourteen days every third month. This schedule results in only four periods each year (after each term of progestin), instead of twelve. The periods may be longer and the bleeding heavier than those produced by monthly periods. This approach may offer enough progestin coverage to protect the endometrium, but more study is needed. One recent study concluded that quarterly progestins (MPA) are, in fact, as safe as taking monthly progestins. Moreover, the study's participants greatly preferred this schedule.

• Estrogens are used continuously with an alternating pattern of progestin use: three days on progestins, three days off, three days on, and so on. A study of this regimen published in *The American Journal of Obstetrics & Gyne-*

cology reported that approximately 90 percent of the 33 women studied had no bleeding during the last twelve months of a twenty-four-month treatment span. Further validation of this regimen's workings is awaited.

• Combined estrogens and progestins are used continuously the first twenty-five days of each month, but are halted for the remainder of the month. Some physicians claim this approach is superior to continuous therapy lasting the entire month because more women reportedly stop bleeding within four months. One to two days of spot bleeding may occur after day 25.

Before choosing a timetable, review the different options with your physician. The more you know what to expect from any one of these schedules, the greater the chances you'll follow through.

A 71-year-old woman who's been on HRT for twenty-five years relates: "I've fine-tuned my own treatment schedule around a five-week cycle: three weeks of oral Premarin alone, followed by one week of Premarin and Provera, followed by one week of nothing. I use a low dose of Permarin—0.3 mg—and 10 mg of Provera. I still get a period. It comes every five weeks."

"Even though I bleed once a month, the schedule I'm on is very manageable and worth putting up with. I take 0.3 mg of Premarin every day and 2.5 mg of Provera on days 1 though 13. My period comes the tenth day of each month—at one o'clock—it's that regular! It lasts for six days, but it's so light that one tampon could last for twelve hours—which I don't do because of the toxic shock syndrome risk."

Wyeth-Ayerst has recently brought to market two new products that package estrogens and progestins together for pill-taking convenience. Prempro has the estrogen and progestin in one pill to be taken daily for continuous combined therapy. Premphase has two separate packages, with estrogens taken for 14 days in one pill and progestins and estrogens for another 14 days in the second pill.

Combining Androgens with Estrogens or Estrogens-Progestins

When prescribed, low-dose androgens are normally taken in tandem with estrogens and estrogen schedules. For instance, if you take estrogens during days 1 through 25 each month, you'll take androgens on the same schedule. Oral tablets that contain both estrogen and testosterone are an increasingly popular administration form, with preparations including full- and half-strength doses. Your doctor may recommend starting with a half-strength dose, judging its effects, and proceeding to a full-strength dose only if needed.

Oral estrogen-androgen combinations include esterified estrogens and methyltestosterone, as well as conjugated estrogens and methyltestosterone. An injected combination makes use of estradiol cypionate and testosterone cypionate.

Estrogen Therapy (Without Progestins)

Postmenopausal women who no longer have a uterus can take unopposed estrogens. Since their uterus is gone, they don't need progestins to prevent endometrial cancer.

If your uterus is intact, you may be able to take estrogens without progestins—if the estrogen dose is low and you have regular endometrial evaluations (at least once a year). An older woman may be the most appropriate candidate for unopposed estrogens, since her uterus is less responsive to estrogen-triggered growth. Also, unopposed estrogens can be a fallback for a woman with a uterus who can't tolerate progestin-induced side effects.

In one study of women with uteri who were on unopposed estrogens, 75 percent of the participants had no bleeding after one year when taking 0.625 mg CEE days 1 through 28. Since women who have a uterus don't often take estrogens alone, because of the greater risk of endometrial cancer, this regimen is not as well known as the other regimens. However, especially when unopposed estrogens are taken on a continuous basis, any bleeding must be evaluated.

For both groups of women—those with an intact uterus and those without—deciding whether to use unopposed estrogens sequentially (days 1 to 25 per month, for instance) or continuously (every day) is a matter of personal choice. Some prefer the sequential approach because it gives them a week away from the bloating, breast tenderness, and other side effects that sometimes accompany estrogen use. Others like continuous therapy because it's easier for them to remember than sequential's stop-and-start schedule.

We need to develop an estrogen whose dose is low enough to protect against heart disease and osteoporosis without stimulating the endometrium or breast tissue. Or it has to be an estrogen that selectively has an effect on the heart and its blood vessels and on the bone but has no effect on endometrial or breast tissue.

Some researchers have suggested that skipping a week

might decrease the risk for cancer, since the body has less exposure to circulating estrogens. But such a hiatus might also allow time for estrogen receptors to become replenished and more receptive to estrogens. Hence, stopping estrogens for a week may yield no benefit. Although neither timetable has been proven better than the other, some researchers hold the opinion that continuous estrogens actually might prove more beneficial to bone and heart.

If you're taking unopposed estrogens for hot-flash relief, stopping the hormone even for only a week may bring their return. Moreover, as estrogens are withdrawn, some women experience headaches, fatigue, and malaise. (These estrogen-associated withdrawal symptoms can also come into play in combined estrogen-progestin sequential therapy.) Continuous estrogen therapy presents no possibility of withdrawal symptoms.

When estrogens are used alone, the doses are the same as those used when progestins and/or androgens are added.

Progestin Therapy

Progestins are commonly taken alone if a woman wants medication to treat postmenopausal hot flashes but is advised against taking estrogens. In such cases, progestins can prove an effective alternative to estrogens, although they can bring undesirable PMS-like side effects. Physi-

> "Two years ago I had a mastectomy. A year later I began getting bad hot flashes. My doctor started me on megestrol acetate [an oral progestin] and the hot flashes disappeared in three days."

cians usually advise a continuous, daily schedule. Progestins aren't commonly used before menopause for hot flashes, because they can cause irregular bleeding.

In the perimenopausal years, progestin-dominant oral contraceptives and HRT progestins can be used to help correct irregular or heavy bleeding and treat endometriosis and endometrial overgrowth.

> "Because my perimenopause was marked by very heavy, very long periods, my doctor put me on oral Provera for the last ten days of each month. It lent to a much more normal cycle."

8

For Hormone Replacement to Work for You, Work with Your Doctor

In the past, many women felt intimidated or shy about discussing menopause and its symptoms with their physicians. On their part, physicians were also apt to keep mention of the "change of life" at arm's length. Any useful dialogue was further stymied by a shortage of information on the subject.

Today, as our knowledge base broadens, a helpful dialogue is opening up between women and their doctors—a trend that needs to be further encouraged. Sponsored by the North American Menopause Society, a survey of 833 women ages 45 to 60 revealed that health-care professionals and their patients still aren't taking the opportunity to discuss menopausal changes as fully as they might. Of the 80 percent of those surveyed who had experienced menopausal symptoms, 33 percent hadn't mentioned their physical symptoms to their doctors. Perhaps more important, many of those surveyed said that their physicians often failed to discuss the menopausal repercussions that concerned them most: osteoporosis, heart disease, and emotional issues. And while many of their physicians addressed hormone replacement therapy, very few made mention of the nonhormonal treatments that are also available for menopausal symptoms and changes. (See the next chapter.)

Knowing you have a doctor who is both knowledgeable about midlife health as well as sensitive to your feelings and questions is an important prerequisite for menopausal and postmenopausal care. A doctor you can trust and easily relate to is essential to good health care at any age, but particularly so during menopause, when sensitive subjects like sexual functioning and genital changes often need to be broached. If your doctor isn't forthcoming with information about menopause, even after your requests, I recommend you find another physician who is more responsive and helpful.

> "When I was 45, I began having terrible night sweats. When I told my doctor I thought it was menopause, he said, 'Oh you're too young. You must be having bad dreams.' That really annoyed me. So I went to a new gynecologist who really listened and put me on the low-dose birth control pill. It reduced my night sweats by about half. Sleeping was much more comfortable."

When you reach menopause, it's wise to consult with a gynecologist or a primary care doctor who will follow your general health-care needs and provide important preventive care (Pap smears and mammograms, for instance), help you address any menopausal symptoms, and monitor hormone replacement therapy, if you decide on that course of treatment. If you require a specialist for another specific problem, your primary doctor's recommendation can often connect you to a specialist in the same circle of care your physician is tied into, facilitating the care you require. With managed health care cited as the wave of the future, a growing trend will be toward a small, central group of doctors providing for your needs.

Numerous menopause clinics have sprouted up across the country. Such clinics can conveniently offer you "one-stop shopping," opening the door to a range of connected specialists. Yet the care available at such centers isn't necessarily better than that offered by a practitioner unaffiliated to such a clinic. Moreover, such a center may provide more tests than are necessary, thus charging more.

Testing Prior to Hormone Replacement Therapy

As mentioned in Chapter 6, several tests taken around the time of menopause can give you a better idea of your health profile and whether or not you should consider replacement hormones. This assessment allows your doctor to make sure you bear no extra risk factors for replacement hormones. It can also help determine which hormone doses and treatment regimen might best serve your particular needs.

More than just a necessary prerequisite for HRT, this pretherapy evaluation gives you an opportunity to come to terms with your health. Menopause represents an excellent time to address health issues that you might have let slip for too long. It's a time when you can take control and potentially avoid some of the health problems so many people encounter in their later years. A face-to-face reckoning with your health may jog you into realizing that it's been six years since you exercised on a regular basis, twenty years since you began smoking, or even longer since you abandoned a thoughtful approach to diet. What better time to set a new agenda!

Necessary Tests before Beginning Hormone Replacement

The tests taken as a prerequisite to hormone replacement therapy vary from doctor to doctor. Those following, however, represent a base core of information collected by most physicians.

- A complete medical history and physical examination, including blood pressure testing, a breast and pelvic exam, and a guaiac test, which checks for blood in the stools or urine, serve as the foundation for any such evaluation.
- Screening tests for cancer include a Pap smear for the detection of cervical cancer and a rectal exam for lower bowel cancer. If you are over 50 and haven't had a mammogram in the past year, you'll need one in order to ensure that no change in breast tissue has occurred.
- A breast cancer screening tool, mammography can detect preclinical cancers. It should be noted, however, that the X-raying of breast tissue doesn't remove the need for breast exams since palpable cancers, ones found through touch, may not appear on mammograms. Mammography reportedly fails to find 20 percent of all breast cancers. Yet the numbers are improving as techniques become more precise. If performed annually after age 50, a mammogram can save lives. Although the debate continues over its effectiveness for women between the ages of

40 and 50, there is evidence that then too it can serve as a life-saving screening tool.

• Your serum cholesterol should be measured to see that it's within normal levels. A cholesterol level exceeding 200 mg/dl should be brought down through diet and exercise, and if significantly higher, by medication. In such cases estrogens can be taken. But your doctor will want to monitor your cholesterol level periodically to make sure it doesn't go up. Oral estrogen therapy potentially can lower total cholesterol by 6 to 10 percent, but in some women with high lipid levels, it occasionally raises cholesterol even higher.

Tests That Are Optional, or Necessary in Certain Situations

• A test to check for sugar in the urine (an indication of diabetes) should be taken if there's a family history of diabetes or if any signs of diabetes are present, such as unexplained weight loss, excessive thirst, or frequent urination.

• I used to perform an endometrial biopsy before prescribing hormones, but it so rarely turned up incidents of hyperplasia that I stopped the practice. The growing trend among physicians is to reserve this oftentimes uncomfortable procedure for cases in which endometrial hyperplasia is suspected. Nonetheless, you may choose to have an endometrial biopsy to rule out any evidence of hyperplasia. If, before going on HRT, you experience unexplained irregular bleeding, you should definitely have an endometrial biopsy.

After HRT is begun, you and your physician should observe your bleeding pattern. Any irregular vaginal bleeding will signal the physician to consider a transvaginal ultrasound, endometrial biopsy, or a *hysteroscopy* (an inspection of the uterine cavity through a telescopic lens) to check for hyperplasia or another condition such as polyps, small tumorlike growths. Increasingly, doctors use a transvaginal ultrasound to monitor the growth of the endometrium, particularly if a woman with an intact uterus is on unopposed estrogens.

• If you have many of the risk factors associated with osteoporosis, or if osteoporosis is a concern for any reason, a bone densitometry measurement can give you and your doctor a clearer sense of the status of your bone mass.

• Although you may elect to have a CA-125 blood test to check for ovarian cancer, this test does not always detect this cancer. ("CA-125" refers to an antigen that appears on ovarian cancer cells.) This blood test does not measure the cancer cells themselves, but a woman's antibody response to the CA-125 antigen. It can produce many false-positive readings (that is, wrongly indicate the disease's presence) if a fibroid or endometriosis is present; moreover, it can fail to find the disease when it is present. This test is most useful after the cancer has been diagnosed, for it can indicate if treatment measures are working.

• Other tests may be called for when indicated. The presence of heart arrhythmia, for instance, may necessitate an electrocardiogram. A thyroid exam may be advisable if you experience chronic fatigue or an excessive loss or gain in weight. Or if anemia is suspected, a *hematocrit*, or blood count, should be taken.

Follow-up Consultation and Office Visits

A month or more after you initiate a hormone replacement regimen, you may need medication adjustments. You may find that 0.625 mg/day of oral conjugated estrogens aren't relieving your hot flashes, for instance, or that a 10 mg oral dose of progestins is triggering excessive anxiety and mood shifts. You should be ready to work with your doctor to find the tailormade regimen that best suits you.

> Mary Riordan, an MGH gynecological nurse, notes: "Sometimes a woman has to try out many different options before she finds the right treatment recipe. We must have tried ten different approaches for one woman whose vaginal dryness had been a problem ever since her menopause. We tried different nonhormonal creams, hormones, even dilators [cones that stretch the vaginal opening]. Finally we hit on what worked: Estrace vaginal cream and Provera. The woman's tissue is clearly improving."

Although doctors' routines vary, most want to hear from their patients within one to two months of starting hormone therapy. It can take this long before doctor and patient are able to assess a woman's overall response to the medication and its effects on shorter-term symptoms. As long as an adequate bank of information has been gathered through pretherapy testing, much of the initial adjustment to a regimen can be done over the phone with your doctor or his or her assistant. It's a good idea to make an office visit four to six months after you've started HRT, at which time you might have an interval medical exam and discuss your bleeding patterns and any side effects. With your doctor's okay, you can then return to your usual schedule of annual checkups, with additional testing (such as a transvaginal ultrasound or endometrial biopsy) when called for. Use your office visits as an opportunity to ask your physician about any new research findings that might pertain to your treatment.

HRT and Drug Interactions

When you take hormone replacement drugs together with other medications, they can sometimes work at cross-purposes. Before you begin HRT, you and your doctor should review whatever other drugs you might be using to ensure against this. Combining HRT with other drugs may change the potency of one drug. Exogenous estrogens taken orally, for instance, may reduce an anticoagulant's protectiveness against blood clotting or alter the effectiveness of a thyroid or antidepressant drug, while a barbiturate can subtract from the intended levels of exogenous estrogens. Higher or lower doses of one medication or the other may be called for. In some cases, you may need to stop taking a particular drug.

Falling Off Your Medication Schedule

As discussed in Chapter 5, many women fail to keep to their medication schedules, skipping days here and there, or going off their medication altogether. If you forget to take your medication, is it bad for you? If you don't keep up with your drug-taking regimen, it isn't going to do you any great harm, but it will obviously reduce the overall effectiveness of your therapy.

If you don't have a uterus and skip a few days of medication, it's not an issue. However, if you skip a few weeks, hot flashes may return; a few months off medication, and vaginal dryness and other symptoms of urogenital atrophy will probably return; after a few years, your bone loss may accelerate to the rate seen directly after menopause. It appears to take several years of estrogen depletion before an associated increased risk for cardiac disease resumes.

If your uterus is intact and you're taking an estrogen-progestin combination, skipping the progestin pills can mean that withdrawal bleeding will start earlier than expected each month. If you skip the progestins but keep using estrogens, you'll be steadily increasing your risk for endometrial hyperplasia and irregular vaginal bleeding.

Alleviating the Side Effects Associated with Progestins

The side effects associated with progestin supplements are usually more noticeable and more of a nuisance than those linked to exogenous estrogens. If you're taking estrogens and progestins "sequentially"—a regimen where you take estrogens for twenty-five days and add progestins for part of the month—then it can be fairly obvious which hormone is responsible for whatever symptoms at a given time. Generally, however, progestins are to blame for the bloating, breast tenderness, irritability, mood changes, and other PMS-like symptoms women may experience when on HRT.

One of the best ways of diminishing these effects is to reduce progestin dosage—from 10 mg to 5 mg, for instance. By some accounts, changing the route of administration—say, from oral to injected progestins—as well as changing the type of synthetic progestin—from a more androgenic progestin to a lesser androgenic progestin—can ease side effects. Yet there is no clear evidence that these alterations work. (As it is, lesser androgenic progestins are widely used for HRT.) Sometimes you may get relief from side effects by switching from an oral synthetic progestin to an oral progesterone, the pure form of the hormone. This is not a sure outcome, however, and oral progesterone itself can be problematic because it isn't always successfully absorbed in the intestinal tract. Also, when the liver metabolizes progesterone, some of the by-products can produce sedativelike action.

> "It's unrealistic to think that one could find a progesterone that has no side effects when, after all, the body's naturally-produced progesterone can account for side effects—namely PMS."

> "For me, finding the right amount of progestins to take took a long time. At first I took too much, and had terrible mood swings and got very bloated. Then, when my doctor decreased my dose, I got signs of hyperplasia. Finally I've found a low-dose combination of estrogens and progestins that works."

Some women find that side effects subside if they change from a sequential regimen for progestins (progestins added to estrogens for seven to twelve days each month, for instance) to a continuous, daily progestin schedule. They can then take less potent progestin doses, since progestin use is spread out over a longer period of time.

Occasionally physicians recommend diuretics for relief from progestin side effects. But this means taking yet another medication, and one that can cause other side effects such as an imbalance of electrolytes, the key compounds that help regulate the body's systems, including the heart. Because of such potential complications, I try to avoid treating one drug's side effects with another drug.

If your troublesome side effects persist, you can stop progestin use and take estrogens alone so long as your endometrial lining is monitored periodically by ultrasound and/or biopsy for excess growth.

Length of Treatment

Many women wonder how long they must remain on hormone therapy. This mostly depends on what you're taking it for. In cases where long-term use is indicated, it also depends on whether you think long-term hormones are advisable for your own personal situation in light of current research findings. Increasingly, the belief is that longer-term hormone therapy is a more effective way to treat vaginal atrophy and protect the heart and bone than shorter-term therapy. Yet this viewpoint is problematic, since longer-term therapy hasn't been thoroughly investigated. Many physicians, however, feel the coast is clear enough—in terms of hormones' recognized risks—to prescribe them long-term. A recommendation is to take hormone therapy one year at a time. Having your health

> "I've been on hormone replacement for sixteen years as a preventive against bone and heart problems. Just recently my doctor and I decided to lower my estrogen dose from 0.625 mg to .3 mg. I feel good about having moved to this lower dose. Taking the higher dose for so long had begun to feel too risky in terms of breast cancer."

reevaluated annually and keeping track of the latest medical findings can help you decide if long-term therapy is useful and/or prudent.

• Treatment for hot flashes: Since untreated hot flashes last an average of six months to three years, you might want to keep up treatment for close to two years, then gradually wean yourself in order to ensure that hot flashes, which are tied to the withdrawal of estrogen, don't recur. If they return even after estrogens have been gradually halted, you may want to resume treatment. However, if they return in a less exaggerated form, you may decide to just grin and bear them, knowing that they're likely to eventually fade away.

• Treatment for vaginal dryness and urogenital atrophy: Unlike hot flashes, vaginal dryness and other symptoms of urogenital atrophy don't diminish over time, but can be lifelong conditions that plague some women more than other women. If these symptoms prove bothersome, long-term estrogen treatment is the best measure. Women fearful of estrogen-related cancers may be more comfortable using the relatively smaller amounts of estrogens in vaginal creams compared to the greater overall doses that usually accompany oral, transdermal or injected estrogens.

• Treatment for heart disease: The data would make you think that the longer you're on estrogens, the better it is for your cardiac health. But there's reason to believe that the women who show these positive results might have been healthier to begin with and therefore don't necessarily present an accurate, representative picture of *all* women's cardiovascular reaction to long-term therapy. Until new research generates more evidence, we can't be absolutely sure of how much heart protection long-term estrogen use provides.

• Treatment for osteoporosis: Beginning estrogen treatment soon after menopause and continuing it for at least seven years appears to preserve bone and reduce fractures. But long-term replacement therapy may protect bone for only so long and may not prevent fractures later in life. If you were to take estrogens for ten years after menopause and then stop, there's some chance that five years later you'd be better protected against fracture than if you hadn't taken hormones at all. Bear in mind, however, that during those five years off therapy, your bone density probably would have declined so rapidly as to make it appear that you'd never taken estrogens.

Part Three

Alternatives to Hormone Replacement

9

Treating Your Symptoms Without Hormones

If your menopausal symptoms or conditions call for treatment, but you have reservations about using supplemental hormones, or they are not advised due to a health concern, there are nonhormonal approaches to consider. These include prescription and nonprescription medications as well as alternative measures. As you'll discover, the medications available are limited, especially given that few such therapies treat menopausal symptoms as effectively as estrogens. This isn't meant as an endorsement for exogenous estrogens to the exclusion of all other treatments, but simply a reflection of current medical and scientific knowledge.

What about alternative options such as herbal remedies, biofeedback, acupuncture, or yoga? Although anecdotally supported, none of these approaches has been rigorously tested. As yet there's no strong consensus in Western medicine as to how well specific alternative approaches work for menopausal symptoms. Eventually, new research emerging from the NIH's Office of Alternative Medicine, the Richard and Hinda Rosenthal Center for Alternative/Complementary Medicine at the College of Physicians and Surgeons, Columbia University, and other new groups should help narrow this gap in our knowledge.

For now, the important message is: If you're seeking an alternative remedy, proceed with care. The fact that alternative therapies are often easily available, yet not yet evaluated by the FDA, necessitates *extra* caution on your part. Moreover, it's imperative to let your doctor know about any alternative therapies you're using, so you both can have a complete picture of your care.

Some professionals suspect that certain alternative therapies "work" only through the placebo effect. "Placebo"—derived from the Latin word *placere,* "to please"—refers to treatment that improves a patient even though the treatment contains no active ingredients that would cause such an improvement. While it's thought to influence the brain, the mechanism behind a placebo remains unknown. As the classic example goes, if you give a sugar pill to a number of patients, 30 percent of them will report feeling better. The duration of the placebo's effectiveness, however, is usually short-lived.

There are, however, other professionals who believe that some of the available alternatives go beyond the placebo effect. "There are enough menopausal women who have had positive experiences [with alternative remedies] to suggest there is something there that is worth studying," says physiologist Fredi Kronenberg, director of the Rosenthal Center. "Women are doing a lot of self-experimenting, and this is helpful because it's giving us guidance for research."

Before settling on either a conventional or alternative nonhormonal approach, explore the choices and weigh whatever information recent reports provide. Also realize that no two women are physiologically alike. What works for a friend's hot flashes might not work for yours. Moreover, just as is true of hormone replacement therapy, it may take a period of trial and error and adjustment before you find a nonhormonal approach that achieves results.

As a side note, some women report that combining small doses of hormones (0.3 mg conjugated estrogens) with other forms of therapy—such as improved nutrition, vitamins, Chinese herbs, or exercise—serves as a useful middle-ground approach for relief of menopausal symptoms and treatment of longer-term conditions.

For Hot Flashes

There are only a small number of proven nonhormonal treatments for menopausal hot flashes. And while they can be effective, they have drawbacks. So unless your symptoms are intolerable, you may want to try waiting out your hot flashes. Remember, hot flashes don't last forever and over time become less frequent and intense. Or you might want to try to overcome them using one or several of the alternative methods discussed later in this section. Because the efficacy of such alternatives on hot flashes isn't proven, bear in mind that if hot flashes subside when an alternative approach is used, it's hard to say if the treatment is actually having an effect, or if your flashes are waning simply because they've run their course.

Prescription Drugs

CLONIDINE

Several antihypertensive drugs can relieve menopausal hot flashes. However, because of such common side effects as fatigue and dizziness, generics such as clonidine may prove impractical for hot flashes. If you have severe flashes but no other recourse for treatment, or if you have hot flashes as well as high blood pressure, these drugs might be appropriate for you. Researchers don't yet know exactly how they subdue flashes, but it's thought that they have a stabilizing effect on the hypothalamus, the body's thermostat.

Shown to alleviate flushing by 30 to 40 percent, clonidine can be used in oral doses of 0.1 and 0.2 mg twice daily. A physician may begin treatment with a lesser dose (0.05 mg twice daily), hoping to both quell hot flashes and keep side effects at bay. Clonidine skin patches are available, which some women find more convenient than pill taking. Inderal, aldomet, and veralipride also are used for menopausal hot flash reduction, as are beta-blockers such as sotalol. None of the above-mentioned drugs has FDA approval for this treatment use.

BELLERGAL

Bellergal, the brand name for a mixture of phenobarbital, belladonna, and ergotamine tartrate, has been shown to reduce hot flashes by 50 percent and has FDA approval for the treatment of menopausal hot flashes. Its downside is that its barbiturate components can cause addiction. Often-reported side effects include dry mouth, fatigue, and depression. Because of its addictive properties, Bellergal isn't usually recommended for hot flashes, and if used should be restricted to the short term.

Note that none of the nonhormonal prescription drugs mentioned in this section is capable of treating vaginal atrophy or osteoporosis.

Vitamins

Through the years, many anecdotal reports have suggested that vitamins E, B, and C can work to suppress hot flashes. No controlled studies have yet confirmed this, however. Kronenberg reported that when she surveyed 251 women who had taken vitamin E specifically for their hot flashes, 27 percent felt the vitamin had brought relief. As Kronenberg and others point out, a well-run controlled study could tell volumes about vitamin E's effect on hot flashes.

Meanwhile, if you want to try quelling your hot flashes with vitamin E, data drawn from the Nurses' Health Study and published in 1993 in *The New England Journal of Medicine* indicates that at the very least you could be doing your coronary-vascular system some good. Researchers found that middle-aged women taking moderate doses of vitamin E (100 IU/day) for over two years had a 40 percent reduced risk of fatal heart attacks and coronary disease than women who didn't take vitamin E supplements. Although the recommended daily allowance for this vitamin is between 12 and 15 IU/day for females, nutritionists often advise supplemental doses of 200 to 800 IU/day for adults. Certain nuts and seeds (pumpkin and sunflower), vegetables and fruits (sweet potato and dried apricots), olive oil, wheat germ, and other foods contain vitamin E, but usually in minimal amounts. Vitamin E is considered fairly nontoxic, although there are occasional reports of headaches, diarrhea, and bleeding problems with very high dosages.

Of the B vitamins, B₆ also has been touted as a hot flash reliever. Some nutritionists also recommend this vitamin for relief from PMS. Anecdotal reports within Western medicine have long held that the B-complex vitamins can help reduce stress. However, whether or not these vitamins can help reduce hot flashes through stress reduction hasn't been examined. The recommended daily allowance for B₆ is 1.6 mg. However, doses of up to 200 mg can be recommended for hot flash treatment. Higher doses run the risk of adversely affecting the nervous system.

While alternative reports sometime make mention of vitamin C as a hot flash soother, there is little information to back this up.

> "When my hot flashes started, my doctor recommended 800 units of vitamin E and 200 mg of B₆. A week later I noticed a real lessening of hot flashes. Some months later I went off E and B₆ because I was taking antibiotics for a bronchial infection and don't like to take too many pills. And you know what? The hot flashes got worse again. I'm convinced these vitamins keep my hot flashes in check."

Body Management

Biofeedback and stress management, relaxation therapies such as yoga, meditation, and deep breathing, as well as plain old exercise are frequently cited ways of relieving hot flashes. But again, a paucity of conclusive evidence makes it hard to judge the true efficacy of these therapies.

EXERCISE

One recent study discovered that hot flashes were less of a complaint among women who exercised regularly at a sports club compared to those who did not. Then again, there are reports that exercise and other situations that make women warmer than usual (hot rooms, hot weather) can worsen hot flashes. Nonetheless, as will be reviewed more fully in this chapter and the next, if you are at menopause's door or through it, you'll be doing your heart, bone, muscle, lungs, digestive tract, mental attitude, and general health a huge favor if you can find time for exercise.

> "When I exercise at home, I use an exercise tape. Invariably I get hot flashes, so I always have a fan going."

BEHAVIORAL MANAGEMENT

In one of the few studies concerned with hot flashes and body management, researchers at the Wayne State University School of Medicine studied 33 women with frequent hot flashes and their responses to deep breathing, muscle relaxation, and brain-wave biofeedback. Deep breathing was associated with a significant reduction in the frequency of hot flashes, while the other two techniques had no effect. This study's small scale makes one reluctant to draw any conclusions. However, the authors speculate that deep breathing somehow works to alter the sympathetic nervous system activity that gives rise to hot flashes.

As Kronenberg points out, self-awareness in general can help a woman cope with hot flashes. If you realize that certain foods trigger flashes, stay away from them. Spicy foods, alcohol, coffee, and other hot drinks, for instance, have been reported to spark hot flashes. If it's apparent that hot flashes occur at a certain time of day, as seems true for some women, being mentally prepared for them can help you override them. Warm rooms, hot days, and hot climates appear to trigger flashes more frequently than cooler temperatures. Keeping in mind that heat can set off flashes, you might dress lightly, sleep with fewer blankets, and generally make it a point to try to stay cooler. If you're aware that stressful situations intensify flashing, anecdotal reports suggest that relaxation techniques such as yoga or meditation can yield results. If your hot flashes are sometimes related to stress, being aware of what's causing stress may help you avoid it and bring relief.

> "Whenever I had meat for dinner, four to six hours later I'd get hot flashes."

Herbal and Other Organic Remedies

Reports that individual herbs and herbal formulas can help combat hot flashes are frequently found in both Western and Eastern literature. The idea that certain herbs might reduce hot flashes and treat other menopausal symptoms and conditions hardly seems far-fetched when you consider how much of our modern pharmacopoeia is based on botanical compounds. Note, for instance, the botanicals used in some licensed hormone products: The root of a wild Mexican yam has been used as a progesterone source for the birth control pill. Soybean is the main active ingredient in Provera, the top-selling HRT progestin in this country, according to its makers.

In regard to many other plants parts and herbs, however, including the various ones mentioned below, it needs to be reiterated that scientific research has yet to prove them effective for menopausal symptoms. I do not prescribe herbal medicines at this time because there are no controlled studies showing their efficacy. Nonetheless, I think it's important to include mention of them in this book since, as future studies evolve, the anecdotal reports provided here and elsewhere may possibly serve as a reference or stepping-off point.

What's generally known is that certain plant compounds can produce progestational and estrogenic effects on humans. The plants and herbs that produce such effects need to be more fully identified, however, along with the specific active agents that provide those effects. What also needs determining is to what extent such botanicals can treat menopausal symptoms and what doses are safe and effective. For now, because of the shortage of hard data, few doctors are in the position to make recommendations.

If you're drawn to your health food store for herbal remedies, it's important to realize that some herbs, just like processed drugs, can exacerbate certain medical conditions and that improper doses can have the wrong effect or no effect at all. In some cases, many different varieties of a particular herb exist (ginseng, for example), each of which may produce a different effect. Add in the fact that there are proliferating numbers of herbal products and product makers, and it can be hard to know which herbal source is most effective. If you're planning to try the herbal approach, it's advisable to review the existing literature as carefully as possible. Make sure that what you're using is at least anecdotally supported and falls within safe parameters. Since natural products aren't regulated by the FDA the same way prescribed drugs are, *precaution is advised.*

Western herbs recommended for menopausal symptoms are apt to be different from those espoused by traditional Chinese medicine. However, herbal practitioners are increasingly drawing from both when prescribing natural products. Two of the herbal roots most frequently cited for hot flash relief are *dong quai* and ginseng. Both substances, alternative practitioners believe, quell flashes by putting mild plant estrogens or plant hormones back into the system, which reportedly help to offset menopause's estrogen deficit. Western herbalists mention numerous other hot flash remedies—in particular, black cohosh, motherwort, caste tree or vitex, chickweed, hawthorn berries, and dandelion. But to reiterate, the effects of these substances have not been validated.

Just as it's not a good idea for a woman with an intact uterus to take pharmaceutical estrogens alone because of the increased risk for uterine cancer, using a single herb for hot flash relief may not be wise, caution many herbalists. In some herbs, the active ingredient is thought to be more progesteronelike; in others, more estrogenlike. "For women with hot flashes who have a uterus, I'm apt to prescribe not only dong quai, an estrogen precursor, but also licorice root, a progesterone precursor," says Tori Hudson, a naturopathic physician at the National College of Naturopathic Medicine in Portland, Oregon. Commonly prepared as tinctures, Western herbs are often prescribed in response to the needs of the whole person, not a specifical condition.

In her book *Menopausal Years: The Wise Woman Way*, herbalist and author Susun Weed provides detail into a range of "herbal allies" for relief from hot flashes, citing the herb motherwort as her personal favorite. Weed also extends beyond botanicals. To manage a bout of flashing, suck on a piece of hard candy, the author advises. Other recommendations by Weed include meditation, a relaxing bath, exercise, and—appropriately—a hand fan.

In traditional Chinese medicine, numerous herbal formulas reportedly can alleviate hot flashes and other menopausal symptoms such as fatigue, headache, and menstrual irregularities. As is increasingly true in the West, herbal formulas resorted to for hot flash relief—such as Two Immortal Decoction, Rehmannia Six Formula, and Geng Nian Formula—aren't employed simply for the relief of an isolated symptom. "In traditional Chinese medicine, a truism is that it's not the condition you treat, but the person," says Barry I. Levine, acupuncturist and herbal prescriber. "Traditionally, the prescribing of these formulas is based on a constellation of signs and symptoms that a person presents." For a woman complaining of hot flashes, a recommended formula might depend upon whether she also displayed an agitated or subdued manner, a pale or pink tongue, robustness or weakness, and numerous other features that indicate her overall health.

Most Chinese formulas are available in pill form and contain natural ingredients long viewed by Eastern cultures as medicinal, such as rehmannia (a yam species), dong quai, oyster shell mineral, white peony (from the tree), and ophiopogon (a variety of asparagus root). Their mixtures have been handed down, generation to generation, for centuries, but they have received little scrutiny from Western medicine.

One of the few double-blind, placebo-controlled studies to investigate the effects of menopausal herbal treatment—with positive results—was led by Tori Hudson and Leanna Standish, also a naturopathic physician, in 1993. When the study began, each of the participants was experiencing one or more menopausal symptoms. While one group was given a placebo, a second group received formulas containing herbs thought to ease menopausal symptoms: glycyrrhiza glabra root (licorice), arctium lappa (burdock), dioscorea villosa (Mexican wild yam), angelica sinensis root (dong quai), and leonurus cardiaca leaf (motherwort). After three months' time, 71 percent of the group on herbs reported relief of all menopausal symptoms in comparison to 17 percent in the placebo group. Relieved symptoms included hot flashes, vaginal dryness, mood changes, and insomnia.

Serving as a small pilot study, the study's major limitation was its small number of participants—13 women. Yet Hudson maintains, "The symptom relief in the group taking herbs was clearly there, well beyond the range of a placebo effect." Nonetheless, before we can safely assume the potential of such substances, much larger studies must be completed.

Just as certain herbs possibly work to reduce menopausal symptoms, diets that regularly contain estrogenic plant components also may help stem hot flashes, some researchers maintain, by adding to estrogen levels in the body. Researchers speculate that some plant factors obtained through diet might also reduce the risk for cancer: by binding to and blocking estrogen receptors, thus diminishing the effects of incoming natural estrogen that otherwise might lead to tumor growth. (Tamoxifen, an estrogenlike compound and a treatment for breast cancer, is thought to work in this manner.)

There is yet a third way, researchers propose, in which consumed plants may regulate estrogen in the body. The fibrous part of plants *(lignin)* may work to absorb excess estrogen in the system, helping to excrete it. Thus there would be less active estrogen in the system to perpetuate cellular overgrowth. On the other hand, if plant-intensive diets are pulling estrogen from the system, what's the effect on bone and other estrogen-nourished body components?

Researchers have barely begun to understand the hormone-regulating effects of plants and herbs, and a clearer reading probably is still many years away. Until then, exercise caution.

Homeopathy

Physicians of homeopathy—the practice of treating a condition with diluted substances that are alleged to create reactions similar to those produced by the illness—maintain that homeopathy also can help relieve a menopausal women's symptoms. Examples of natural substances used include plant extracts, minerals, bacteria, venoms, and other animal products. For instance, a homeopathic preparation of sepia—the ink secreted from a squid—can work to subdue hot flashes, according to homeopathic practitioners. It's also been reported that iodine can reduce mood swings and anxiety, and phosphorous can lessen heavy perimenopausal bleeding. While homeopathy has aroused considerable skepticism in some quarters, in a report to the journal *Lancet,* Dr. Carol D. Berkowitz of Harbor/UCLA Medical Center in Torrance, California, appealed to physicians to keep an open mind with respect to this alternative practice. "The principle that small doses of potentially harmful substances can augment a healthy response is no stranger to accepted medical practices," wrote Berkowitz, who points to substances used to desensitize allergic reactions as a good example of this. For instance, Berkowitz notes, when small amounts of venom are used for a bee sting, it causes antibodies to develop, desensitizing the person against an allergen and allergic response. Similarly, vaccines using weakened or dead germs work to build up the body's defenses.

Bear in mind, however, that in regard to homeopathy, the research hasn't taken place. There is no way of yet knowing if, or to what extent, it is useful for menopausal symptoms.

Acupuncture

Few Western reports suggest that acupuncture is useful for subduing hot flashes; fuller evidence supports its benefit for other menopause-related symptoms. However, one recent noteworthy Swedish study of 21 women with menopausal hot flashes did find that acupuncture significantly reduced symptoms, with its effects lasting at least three months after treatment had ended. "Actually, the use of acupuncture to treat menopausal problems may be new to Western medicine, but it has long been used in China, Japan, and other countries, both alone and in combination with herbs and other remedies," Fredi Kronenberg of Columbia University comments in an editorial that appeared with the above-mentioned study in the journal *Menopause*. Some alternative practitioners contend that acupuncture affects aspects of the nervous system that give rise to hot flashes.

Research is gradually revealing that acupuncture stimulates nerve points under the skin that trigger the release of endorphins, natural analgesics found in the spinal cord,

> "When dong quai didn't work for my hot flashes, I turned to acupuncture. It really seems to have kept them in check."

> "I was getting my period as frequently as every fifteen to twenty days. Acupuncture worked to lengthen the time between my periods to thirty days."

brain, and pituitary gland. There's quite a bit of solid evidence that acupuncture can help relieve perimenopausal heavy and erratic menstrual bleeding as well as pain and headache associated with menstruation. There are frequent references, too, to acupuncture's positive effects on insomnia and stress.

For Urogenital Atrophy

Compared to the scant number of *proven* nonestrogen options for hot flash relief, proven nonhormonal approaches for revitalizing vaginal tissue are more numerous. Yet, unlike hot flashes, for some women vaginal atrophy may be a long-term disorder and its treatment can be limited by age-driven factors.

Nonhormonal Vaginal Moisturizers

Several over-the-counter vaginal lubricants can help women overcome vaginal dryness, painful intercourse, and painful urination due to estrogen depletion. You should make sure that the moisturizer you choose is water soluble, since those that aren't (petroleum jelly, for instance) create a moisture barrier that works against lubrication. Certain of these products are used only at the time of intercourse, while others are designed for more continuous relief of vaginal dryness.

Nonhormonal creams can relieve vaginal dryness more

rapidly than estrogen creams. But since they contain no estrogens, they won't stimulate a cellular buildup of vaginal tissue over time. Therefore, for a continuous reduction of vaginal dryness, you'll need to keep reusing the recommended dosage continuously. In comparison, estrogen cream doses can often be reduced as vaginal dryness abates. Over-the-counter vaginal moisturizers don't change the underlying condition of vaginal cells. Therefore don't expect them to treat more deep-seated atrophic disorders such as incontinence or muscular weakness—conditions that may not even respond to replacement estrogens. Also, vaginal lubricants aren't as effective as vaginal estrogens in controlling urinary tract infections. Yet they can help maintain a pH level that thwarts infection.

Most over-the-counter vaginal moisturizers work short-term, at the time of use. Polycarbophil, the active ingredient in the product Replens, represents a novel effort toward continuous treatment of vaginal dryness. Its bio-adhesive delivery system draws water out of cells into the vaginal area. Hence the body's own fluids lend to continuous lubrication. Being the Rolls-Royce of vaginal moisturizers, Replens is on the expensive side. It's usually used three times a week. Other effective over-the-counter moisturizers include Astroglide (a gel) and Lubrin (a suppository).

Behavioral Therapy for Incontinence

PELVIC EXERCISES

If you have incontinence caused by weakened pelvic floor muscles, strengthening those muscles through exercise can improve bladder control. For women with stress incontinence, tensing the pubococcygeal muscles located around

the vaginal opening and anus for a set number of repeti-
tions each day can bring positive results within eight
weeks, even for older women. Exercises for incontinence
are often referred to as the Kegel exercises, named after
Dr. Arnold Kegel, the surgeon who developed this therapy
in the 1950s. To get a feel for those muscles that support
the urethra, uterus, and rectum, try to stop the flow of
urine when you relieve your bladder. Doing your Kegels
faithfully can restore your pelvic floor muscles enough
that a sneeze or heavy lifting won't cause urination. A key
point in this training—which can also improve some cases
of urge incontinence—is that it can work for the properly
selected patient so long as exercises are done regularly and
consistently. You should consult a health-care professional
for a detailed exercise program.

Kegel exercises in combination with low-dose estrogens
can prove to be a particularly effective therapy for incontinence. "Exogenous estrogens can replenish the cellular
surface of the urinary opening, the base of the bladder,
and the lining of the urinary passage, while exercise can
build up muscles, providing for the closure of the bladder"
so that urine will not leak out, explains MGH gynecologist Dr. George S. Richardson.

BIOFEEDBACK

Several studies report that biofeedback that focuses on the
workings of the pelvic floor muscles can help improve
bladder control in some women. A transvaginal sensor inserted into the vagina and connected to a computer and
monitor measures muscular activity, showing a woman
just how effectively she is contracting her pelvic muscles.
The monitor presents instant feedback as to which muscles need more training and strengthening.

VAGINAL CONES

These tampon-shaped, hard plastic weights are, in essence, a type of biofeedback technique that can help a woman strengthen her pelvic-floor muscles to achieve better bladder control. Once a cone is inserted into the vagina, a woman walks around and tries to hold it in by tensing appropriate muscles. If the cone slides out, she is tensing the wrong muscles and needs further pelvic training.

BLADDER TRAINING

Bladder training that aims at determining how often a woman needs to urinate and increasing the intervals between voiding can also aid bladder control.

> "Every day I do a combination of Kegels and bladder drills, and in a year and a half my stress incontinence and frequency have improved tremendously. For Kegels, I squeeze the vaginal muscles ten times in a row at least six times a day. When I first started the bladder drills, I was having to urinate every fifteen or twenty minutes. The first goal was to try not to go to the bathroom for thirty minutes. At first I leaked, but then I made it through thirty minutes. That was a real triumph. Then I worked up to an hour, then two hours, then three hours. Now, sometimes I can even go for four hours without urinating. I still have stress incontinence, but I usually notice it only when I've got a cold and have a bad cough."

New Therapeutic Devices for Incontinence

FUNCTIONAL ELECTRICAL STIMULATION

This promising approach, which makes use of a vaginal probe, delivers short bursts of electrical current through the vaginal wall to pelvic muscles, causing pelvic muscles to contract and, over time, strengthen. Some reports state that electrical stimulation can significantly reduce incontinence, although the full benefits of this technique need further review. The procedure is usually performed on a daily basis for several weeks.

Collagen Implants

Recently approved by the FDA for specific causes of stress urinary incontinence, this procedure involves the use of collagen, a protein found in humans and animals. When collagen is injected into tissue around the urethra, it can build up tissue bulk. This provides more pressure around the urethra so that if intra-abdominal pressure increases because of a cough or sneeze, it will be counteracted by the collagen, and thus urine will not leak out. This technique reportedly has a 50 to 75 percent success rate.

Medications and Surgery for Incontinence

Although no safe and effective drugs are available for relief from stress incontinence, a few medications can improve urge incontinence for certain women. The antidepressant imipramine, for example, relaxes the bladder, which can serve to make the pressure of the urethra greater than the pressure in the bladder, preventing leakage. Imipramine's side effects (dry mouth, dizziness), however, may limit its use. Ditropan (brand name), an antispasmodic, is also used to treat incontinence, although users may experience diarrhea, drowsiness, blurred vision and other side effects.

If stress incontinence is severe, many different types of surgery can be attempted. The general goal is to restore the structural relationship between the urethra, urthrovesical junction, bladder, and other pelvic organs. However, surgery can also create new bladder-related disorders, including urge incontinence and voiding problems. If surgery is undertaken, the drawbacks that might arise may still seem more manageable than what a woman was experiencing beforehand.

Diet for Urogenital Conditions

As recently demonstrated, century-old wives' tales concerning alternative therapies shouldn't be written off. Cranberry juice's long-rumored ability to curb urinary tract infections took on new credibility with a report published in March 1994. In the first large-scale controlled study of its kind, researchers from the Harvard Medical School studied 153 women over age 65. One randomly assigned group drank ten ounces a day of a low-cal cranberry juice cocktail. A second randomly-assigned group imbibed the same quantity of a nonjuice taste-alike. After six months, the cranberry juice drinkers had a 58 percent reduction in their risk of having bacteria and white blood cells (a sign of infection) in their urine compared to the placebo group.

The juice drinkers' urine was no more acidic than the nonjuice drinkers', dispelling the notion that cranberry juice's acidity is what smites harmful bacteria. The researchers instead theorized that cranberry juice may make it harder for bacteria to stick to the bladder's inner wall and helps flush out bacteria in the urine. Therefore, while cranberry juice can help prevent infections, it "shouldn't be used as a substitute for antibiotics with a urinary tract infection that is producing symptoms," writes Dr. Jerry Avorn, the study's lead author. Along with cranberry, other members of the Vaccinium family—for example, blueberry and bilberry—may also cut down on urinary tract infections, it's been suggested.

As for anecdotal reports that cranberry juice can reduce incontinence, no confirming studies exist. However, other foods are thought to influence incontinence. Spices and spicy foods can irritate urgency problems, as can caffeine, alcohol, and acidic foods like tomatoes and citrus fruits. Smoking is thought to substantially raise the risk of developing incontinence by decreasing a woman's total circulating estrogens, which can worsen urogenital atrophy. The coughing associated with smoking also can weaken pelvic muscles that support bladder function.

If menopause's estrogen depletion can promote unhealthy urogenital bacteria, are vaginal yeast infections also more prevalent in the postmenopausal years? And if so, is it true that yogurt helps ward off yeast overgrowth? Actually, yeast infections happen more readily in estrogen's presence, not its absence. Researchers report a higher incidence of vaginal yeast overgrowth in menstruating women than in postmenopausal women or young girls.

Another surprise: When yeast overgrowth is a problem, yogurt may not be the preventive it's trumped up to be. In 1992 a study that found that women who consumed yogurt fended off yeast infections raised a lot of interest. Yet, some researchers now believe that the study was flawed and that yogurt doesn't necessarily keep yeast overgrowth at bay. Nonetheless, there are still those who swear by yogurt, maintaining that a cup consumed each day or a few tablespoons of plain yogurt inserted daily into the vagina is an effective preventive tactic, so long as the yogurt contains active bacteria cultures.

Alternative suggestions for vaginal dryness and itching, bladder control, and urinary tract infections form a long list. But, again, a lack of hard supporting evidence makes any evaluation of these recommendations difficult. Suggestions for dry vaginal tissue are particularly numerous and include comfrey, slippery elm, vitamin E suppositories, the herb calendula, and progesterone cream derived from the wild yam. Herbalist Susun Weed notes that, in particular, dong quai and motherwort can serve as effective relievers of dryness. For a fast-acting topical treatment, she recommends inserting a capsule of acidophilus into the vaginal all the way up to the cervix. Since acidophilus can bring quick results, says Weed, capsules are often used on a daily basis for a short time, then more occasionally after that.

The stimulation of sex itself can help vaginal tissue stay moist. For postmenopausal women not on estrogens, who haven't had sex for a long time, self-dilation (stretching the vaginal opening with your fingers) can prepare vaginal tissue for renewed activity.

For Bone Loss

Generally it's a promising time for research into nonestrogen treatments aimed at either preventing bone loss or stimulating new bone formation. Many possibilities are being explored, with the goal of finding a therapy that substantially activates bone growth. While currently prescribed therapies, including estrogens, *slow* bone loss, none offered thus far consistently and safely produces an *increase* in bone. Finding a treatment that could stimulate bone growth would be a major step toward strengthening the skeleton and avoiding osteoporosis.

Note: Included in this section are treatments that use

hormones derived from the thyroid and parathyroid glands. These hormones aren't considered "hormone replacement" therapies since they aren't replacing ovarian-made hormones. Their use does not appear to create the cancer-related risks cited for exogenous estrogens.

Prescription Drugs

CALCITONIN

A hormone made by the thyroid gland, calcitonin is known to inhibit bone resorption, the process by which bone is broken down and reabsorbed in the body. There's indication that it also regulates calcium metabolism. When used as a treatment, calcitonin has been shown to slow bone loss and may improve bone density. However, it hasn't been shown to decrease fractures in post-menopausal women the way replacement estrogens have been shown to do. The current feeling is that this treatment measure can be most beneficial for women who have a high bone turnover with rapid bone loss.

Usually given by injection, calcitonin may produce flushing, nausea, and dizziness. Less than 10 percent of patients experience these effects which, on average, are mild and transient. Moreover, side effects can be minimized by taking the drug at bedtime. Calcitonin, which for treatment purposes is derived from fish calcitonin, comes at a high cost. If taken for a year at a dose of 100 units/day, it can run as high as $3,000. However, lower doses can be useful—for example, 100 units taken three times a week. A calcitonin nasal spray has been approved by the FDA to treat osteoporosis. It is sprayed in one nostril one day and the other nostril the other day.

Replacement estrogens and calcitonin are the only medications approved by the FDA for the treatment of bone loss. Unless they get the nod from the FDA for the treatment of bone, other therapies—including those below—should be considered experimental, advises Dr. David M. Slovik, an MGH bone specialist.

BISPHOSPHONATES

This class of medicines was originally approved to reduce the bone breakdown and abnormal bone repair seen in patients with Paget's disease. The bisphosphonates are synthetic compounds made out of phosphorous and carbon. When incorporated into bone, they inhibit bone resorption and may reduce the vertebral fracture rate. While these compounds can work as a successful short-term therapy for postmenopausal bone loss, their longer-term effects on osteoporosis aren't yet known.

The bisphosphonate most in use for treating bone disorders is etidronate (generic name), a drug which has federal approval for the treatment of Paget's disease and high levels of calcium in the blood due to cancer *(hypercalcemia)*. Initial studies suggest that an effective regimen consists of taking etidronate daily (400 mg) for two weeks every three months, with calcium (1,000 to 1,500 mg) taken daily when the drug isn't being taken.

Given by mouth, the bisphosphonates are very poorly absorbed. An empty stomach will maximize absorption, according to Slovik. When used for bone loss treatment, these drugs so far have evidenced no significant side effects and perhaps could end up costing less than calcitonin. All in all, this therapy may have a promising future, say researchers. Several new potent bisphosphonates which are taken daily are currently being investigated and will soon be available.

Fosamax

A new drug called Fosamax (alendrinate) shows promise in treating women who already have osteoporosis. In a five-year study, women with low bone density were able to increase their bone density with daily doses of Fosamax, which is similar to the etidronates described above. Since it is poorly absorbed from the intestines, Fosamax must be taken on an empty stomach, so doctors recommend that patients take it first thing in the morning with a glass of water and then wait a half hour before eating anything. The major side effect is esophageal ulceration, so patients shouldn't lie down directly after taking the medication. Further studies will be needed to determine whether Fosamax is effective in preventing osteoporosis in women who do not already have it, or whether it would be more effective when combined with estrogens for women with severe osteoporosis.

Parathyroid Hormones

Also still in the process of being investigated, this treatment carries the unique potential of *activating* new bone growth, according to researchers, unlike other available treatments, which mostly retard bone loss. Parathyroid hormone is produced in four small glands located behind the thyroid gland. When low doses of parathyroid hormone are administered intermittently by once-a-day injections, the result is the stimulation of bone-forming cells *(osteoblasts)* and an increase in bone mass. In human studies, this approach has consistently resulted in significant increases in trabecular bone (the spongy, inner part of bone) of the spine, according to Slovik. Few changes in cortical bone (the outer, more dense part of bone) have been observed. Still, many questions about this approach need answering, especially concerning long-term use. Moreover, no double-blind controlled studies have yet affirmed this drug's efficacy.

A study by MGH and Brigham and Women's Hospital researchers recently showed that parathyroid hormone injections can help prevent the bone loss caused by GnRH agonists—drug treatments that slow the growth of endometriosis and fibroids. A problem with current GnRH-agonist therapy is that it usually isn't given for longer than six months because of its negative impact on bone. These new results hold out hope for a way of providing more long-lasting GnRH-agonist therapy.

THIAZIDE DIURETICS

Although research has shown that thiazide diuretics can reduce calcium excretion and slow bone loss, their use isn't recommended as a primary treatment for post-menopausal bone loss at this time. Too few large clinical trials leave an inexact picture of their effects on bone loss. Slovik advises, "They should only be employed for bone therapy in special situations, notably when a woman is excreting a large amount of calcium in her urine."

TAMOXIFEN

An increasingly used treatment for breast cancer, the drug tamoxifen works like an estrogen in that it can bind to an estrogen breast receptor. But unlike a pure estrogen, it can block estrogenic activity in the cells it attaches to; hence its use in breast cancer therapy.

Interestingly enough, early studies have reported that when breast cancer patients are treated with tamoxifen, it appears to decrease bone loss. Paradoxically, here is a drug that seems to detract from estrogen activity in the breast, yet produces estrogenlike activity on bone. Researchers are currently trying to decipher if tamoxifen might be an appropriate therapy for osteoporosis. "Until more data are available, tamoxifen should not be administered for any other reason but its approved indications," cautions Slovik.

Dietary Treatments

FLUORIDE

Many Americans get fluoride in the water they drink or in the increasing number of marketed products that contain fluoride—toothpastes, mouth rinses, and fluoride gels, for example. The amounts put into the water by various cities and towns have been shown to lessen tooth decay. There is also some evidence that fluoride-treated water is associated with a lower rate of bone fracture.

The concept of using larger amounts of sodium fluoride to treat bone loss in postmenopausal women remains controversial. Fluoride can trigger new bone formation and inhibit bone loss. But there's evidence that the bone that forms isn't always normal, healthy bone, but instead is more vulnerable to fracture. Moreover, fluoride may strengthen some bones at the expense of others. Larger doses particularly have more negative effects, studies reveal. (The smaller amounts added to water consumed by the public, however, are deemed safe.) Up to one-half of those treated with fluoride experience nausea, gastritis, joint pain, and other troublesome side effects. The medical consensus is that fluoride's long-term use, the potency of its varying doses, and newer fluoride forms all require further analysis. For now, fluoride shouldn't be used as a bone-loss treatment, maintains Dr. Donald Deraska,

MGH endocrinologist. Meanwhile, a new slow-release form of fluoride with the potential to stimulate strong bone formation is undergoing investigation.

Calcium

As calcium gets incorporated into bone, it plays an active role in creating strong, durable bone tissue. One would think, then, that calcium supplements taken around menopause might help stop the rapid bone loss that has been observed during the years directly after menopause. This doesn't appear to be the case, researchers have discovered. "The bone loss that happens right after menopause is such an accelerated loss that calcium cannot preserve premenopausal bone density levels, but it can decrease bone loss to some extent," explains Mary Carey, director of the Graduate Program in Dietetics at MGH Institute of Health Professions.

Therefore calcium is not considered a treatment for menopausal bone loss. This doesn't mean that women shouldn't be taking calcium at this point in their lives, reiterates Carey. Calcium can slow the loss somewhat and may be fortifying bone's durability. Moreover, if estrogens are being taken for bone loss, the addition of supplemental calcium can enable women to take lower doses of estrogen. Women who have reservations about taking estrogen yet need bone therapy may feel better about taking, for example, 0.3 mg/CEE/day plus calcium rather than the higher dose of 0.625/CEE/day without calcium. An estrogen-calcium combination not only can retard bone loss but also can lower the future risk of fracture.

Even though you shouldn't depend on calcium to stop immediate menopausal bone loss, getting enough calcium

Table 3. Top Sources of Calcium

Food Item	Serving Size	Calcium Content (mg)	Calories
Milk			
Whole	8 oz	291	150
Skim	8 oz	302	85
Yogurt (with added milk solids)			
Plain, low fat	8 oz	415	145
Frozen, fruit	8 oz	240	223
Cheese			
Mozzarella, part skim	1 oz	207	80
Muenster	1 oz	203	105
Cheddar	1 oz	204	115
Ricotta, part skim	4 oz	335	190
Cottage, low-fat (2% fat)	4 oz	78	103
Ice Cream, Vanilla (11% fat)			
Hard	1 cup	176	270
Soft serve	1 cup	236	375
Ice Milk, Vanilla			
Hard (4% fat)	1 cup	176	185
Soft Serve (3% fat)	1 cup	274	225
Fish and Shellfish			
Sardines, canned in oil drained, *including bones*	3 oz	372	175
Salmon, pink, canned, *including bones*	3 oz	167	120
Vegetables			
Bok choy, raw	1 cup	74	9
Broccoli, cooked, drained, from raw	1 cup	136	40
Soybeans, cooked, drained from raw	1 cup	131	235
Collards, cooked, drained from raw	1 cup	357	65
Turnip greens, cooked, drained from raw (leaves and stems)	1 cup	252	30
Tofu	4 oz	108*	85
Almonds	1 oz	75	165

* The calcium content of tofu may vary depending on processing methods. Tofu processed with calcium salts can have as much as 300 mg calcium per 4 oz. Often, the label or the manufacturer can provide more specific information.

Source: National Osteoporosis Foundation.

through diet and supplements (if needed) before and after menopause remains important for several reasons. If you nourish your bone with adequate calcium before menopause, it might be like putting money in the bank; your bone density might be greater, resulting in less signs of bone breakdown after menopause. Also, adequate calcium before and after menopause may help curtail age-related bone breakdown. It's been shown that during the years after menopause's period of accelerated bone loss, calcium supplements can in fact slow bone loss in older women, especially those who aren't getting enough calcium from food.

The National Osteoporosis Foundation recommends 1,000 mg/day of dietary calcium for premenopausal adult women as well as for postmenopausal women who take estrogens. If you're postmenopausal and don't take estrogens, your body may need as much as 1,500 mg/day of calcium. This increase is advised because once levels of ovarian-made estrogens decline, the body doesn't absorb calcium as well as it did.

Certain dairy foods are deemed the best sources of calcium, especially milk, cheese, and yogurt. Certain seafood (shrimp, oysters, canned sardines, and salmon with bones) and vegetables (broccoli, collards, watercress, parsley, and turnip greens, for example) also contain high quantities of this mineral. As for other nondairy foods, calcium turns up in surprising places. It's present in fairly substantial quantities in tofu (as long it's made with calcium sulfate), certain nuts (such as almonds, pecans, and Brazil nuts) as well as molasses and maple sugar. (See Table 3.) Kelp, it turns out, is one of the most calcium-rich plants available. While kelp isn't on most dinner menus, it's available in supplemental form. Getting into the habit of having one calcium-rich food a day—say a cup of low-fat yogurt (400 mg/calcium) or two glasses of skim milk (600 mg)—can help you achieve the recommended daily intake.

For some women, an adequate dietary intake of calcium can be hampered by the inability to digest milk sugar, a condition known as lactose intolerance. If the consumption of milk products routinely causes bloating, intestinal gas, or diarrhea, you are probably lactose intolerant. The condition is caused by a deficiency of *lactase*, an enzyme which helps break down lactose, milk's primary sugar. In the absence of this enzyme, lactose becomes fermented, producing carbon dioxide, which causes the discomfort. In adulthood, the enzyme deficiency results in symptoms in 10 to 15 percent of white Americans, 70 to 90 percent of blacks and Asians. It isn't known why certain populations are particularly vulnerable.

As long as you're aware you have this condition—and most women do—it needn't be an obstacle to calcium intake. Many people who are lactose intolerant can consume small amounts of milk products and should try to do so. Drinking small quantities of milk several times a day can help reduce unwanted symptoms. Many products are available today that can ease the woes of lactose intolerance, including lactose-reduced milk.

Most nutrition guides warn against various foods that hinder calcium absorption: phosphorus-containing cola drinks; oxalic acid that is found in certain foods such as Swiss chard, beet greens, spinach, rhubarb, and the cocoa bean (hence chocolate); excess dietary fiber; and excess protein. These are the culprits regularly mentioned. However, it would take very large quantities of these foods to interfere with calcium absorption, maintains Carey at the MGH. "Most people don't eat huge amounts of these foods," said Carey. "For instance, eating too much fiber usually isn't an issue. Most people, as it is, don't eat enough fiber." Also, whether or not phosphorous is bad for bone is a controversial issue, according to Carey. The phosphorous in cola drinks might be less of a problem than the fact that such drinks are replacing more beneficial liquids, such as milk or water. The observation that caffeine reduces dietary calcium by increasing its urinary excretion also needs validation, some researchers believe.

As long as your food intake is within range of the FDA's food pyramid's dietary guidelines, you shouldn't have a problem with calcium-robbing foods, maintains Carey.

Table 4. Calcium Preparations

PREPARATION	CALCIUM PERCENTAGE	CALCIUM (MG) PER TABLET	YEARLY COST* FOR 1,000 MG/DAY
Calcium carbonate	40		
Caltrate		600	$ 108
Oyster shell (generic)		250, 500, 600	$ 40
Os-Cal		250, 500	$ 108
Tums-Ex		300	$ 55
Calcium Rich Rolaids		220	$ 53
Calcium phosphate			
Posture	40	600	$ 115
Calcium lactate (650 mg)	13	85	$ 350
Calcium gluconate (975 mg)	9	90	$ 522
Calcium citrate	8		
Citracal		200, 315	$ 162

* Discount retail price

This list shows how available preparations can vary greatly in the percentage of elemental calcium they contain, the number of milligrams of calcium per tablet, and annual cost. With tablets containing less elemental calcium, you may need to take two or more tablets to get the calcium you need.

Source: *Menopause Management*, May 1993, and Ettinger, B. "Postmenopausal Osteoporosis." In Bardin W., ed., *Current Therapy in Endocrinology and Metabolism.* St. Louis: Mosby-Year Book Inc., 1994:596–600.

(For a review of those guidelines, refer to the next chapter.) A much more important issue is that even if you eat wisely, you may not be consuming enough dietary calcium.

If you're postmenopausal and not on calcium supplements, there's a good chance that your calcium intake is below, perhaps far below, the recommended 1,500 mg/day of calcium. (An intake of 1,500 mg/day is equivalent to five glasses of milk.) A Nationwide Food Consumption Survey found that the average intake of calcium among all Americans is less than 800 mg/day. Some researchers suspect that, postmenopausally, women often take in as little or less than 500 mg/day. Women are apt to shun dairy products because of their fat content. Yet since the body needs some dietary fat, as well as calcium, dairy products aren't necessarily the foods to avoid. Fatty meats or fried

---

"My bone density is what it should be for my age," notes a 66-year-old woman. "But I'm susceptible to fractures, so each day I drink two and a half glasses of skim milk, have one yogurt, and take a Tums 500-mg calcium supplement three times a day."

---

foods should be the first to go. Moreover, skim milk and nonfat cheeses and yogurt will give you the calcium you need without the fat.

When your dietary intake of calcium is insufficient, supplemental calcium can make up the difference. Be aware, however, that a multivitamin doesn't necessarily contain calcium. Calcium, a mineral, may require a separate purchase. Calcium carbonate and calcium citrate are the most common supplements available. Although calcium carbonate can cause bloating, intestinal gas, and constipation, taken with meals, this supplement is likely to be better absorbed and give rise to fewer symptoms. Calcium citrate, on the other hand, should not be taken with meals. Because different forms of calcium should be taken at different times to ensure optimal absorption, read any supplement's instructions carefully. It's also advisable to consult a physician when taking calcium.

A good rule of thumb, according to Carey, is to spread calcium supplement use throughout the day, taking no more than 500 mg at a time, since too much ingested all at once can produce kidney stones in some people. Supplemental calcium is also available in fortified cereals, breads, juices, and the antacid Tums or its generic equivalents. Many women take tablet supplements because it's easier to keep track of how much calcium they're consuming.

The overconsumption of calcium, as well as of vitamin D, can lead to *hypercalcemia* and *hypercalciuria*. The former refers to too much calcium in the blood, which in severe cases can lead to muscle failure, confusion, and kidney failure. The latter, which often accompanies hypercalcemia, occurs when there's so much calcium in the urine that it causes kidney stones. As mentioned, taking calcium throughout the day can avoid this latter risk. All told, however, most women are in danger of getting far too little calcium rather than far too much, particularly after menopause.

Vitamin D

You can load yourself with calcium every day and still be calcium deficient if you don't have enough vitamin D in your system. Vitamin D helps the small intestine absorb calcium and paves the way for calcium's uptake by bone. Many women receive ample amounts of vitamin D from sun exposure and a balanced diet, which can include vitamin-D fortified milk. Other high-calcium foods are also fortified with vitamin D, including cereals and instant breakfasts.

During summer, approximately twenty to thirty minutes of sun a day provides adequate amounts of vitamin D. But don't count on winter sun. In the north, even many hours' worth of total-body exposure to winter sun—hardly a likely scenario—converts only negligible amounts of vitamin D. The sun has to be direct and intense for its ultraviolet rays to facilitate the conversion of vitamin D precursors in the skin to the active vitamin. Since vitamin D stays in the body for a long time, women in northern regions who receive plenty of exposure to summer sun often can get through winter without D supplements, although some nutritionists recommend supplements be taken during winter months. If you're over 60, it's a good idea to take a daily multivitamin that includes the recommended 400 international units of vitamin D, especially since your skin is thinner and your body is less able to make the vitamin. Note that sunscreens, which block out ultraviolet rays, can lower the conversion of vitamin D.

If you don't get out in the sun, eat a less well balanced diet, or are prone to a vitamin D deficiency, you may require supplements in order to meet the daily recommended 400 IU of vitamin D.

The possibility of using a potent form of vitamin D to directly treat osteoporosis is under investigation. Although some reports suggest that synthesized metabolites of D can reduce bone loss, the findings in this regard have been inconclusive.

ALTERNATIVE DIETARY THERAPIES FOR BONE LOSS

Given that a range of vitamins and minerals reportedly support healthy bone, it's reasonable to think that many

Figure 9. Fracture Sites

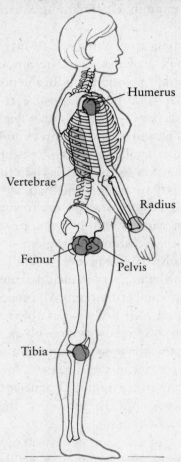

The most common sites of fracture related to postmenopausal (type 1) osteoporosis are marked by light-gray circles and those related to senile (type 2) osteoporosis are marked by dark-gray circles. Postmenopausal osteoporosis refers to estrogen-related bone loss. Senile osteoporosis is age-related.

Illustration: Harriet Greenfield.

substances from land and sea can help nourish bone. Among those recommended by naturalists are various seaweeds (hijiki and kombu, for example), land weeds (dandelion and nettles), the herb horsetail, microcrystalline hydroxyapatite (a whole-bone extract), and calcium-rich oatstraw. Kelp is one of the most calcium-rich plants in nature. Anecdotal reports also suggest that progesterone cream derived from wild yams can slow bone loss and reduce fractures.

Some nutritionists claim that so much attention is devoted to calcium and vitamin D that the importance of many other bone-nourishing micronutrients—such as magnesium, boron, silicon, zinc, copper, and vitamins C and K—get overlooked. Yet not enough information has been amassed to know for sure what role numerous compounds and trace elements might play in bone maintenance. A balanced diet, however, should provide you with most of them.

Exercise for Osteoporosis

Researchers speculate that our ancestors probably had thicker, stronger bones than we have today, especially those of us living in industrialized nations. Rising rates of fractures also suggest that something about modern life is detrimental to healthy bone. While diet may be one contributor to bone loss, researchers theorize that inactivity and lack of exercise may be the straw that is breaking the camel's back.

Accumulating evidence keeps underscoring the same point: *Regular exercise keeps bone primed and helps prevent bone deterioration.* How it accomplishes this feat is still being examined. Exercise may be directly affecting bone by stimulating metabolic hormones that influence such growth. There's considerable evidence that exercise also indirectly affects bone by applying force on the muscles connected to bone. The more a muscle is moved, the more electromagnetic resistance develops between muscle and bone, and the more bone stays primed in response to that stress. When bone isn't stressed by muscle, it can break down rapidly.

MGH bone specialists offer the following familiar advice for postmenopausal women: Use it or lose it. Any physical activity is better than none at all. However, while researchers agree that exercise helps reduce the rate of bone loss and fracture, whether or not it can build up bone significantly depends upon whom you ask. Some researchers say that even the most optimistic studies find that exercise augments bone density only minimally, by no more than 3 to 5 percent. Others report considerably higher bone density measurements in women who exercise—even older women—compared to those who don't. Yet "that doesn't prove exercise is responsible [for significant bone increases]," notes MGH's Dr. Robert M. Neer. In some cases, it could be that those who are exercising more are eating more, hence providing more nutrients for the bone-building process.

When bone density increases, to whatever degree, the greatest buildup occurs in those locations most influenced by exercise. For instance, a squash player's racquet arm will contain denser bone than his or her free arm. In the United States, where people are predominantly right-handed, the population has 1 percent more bone mass in the right arm than the left. When exercise contributes to bone buildup, the body appears to reach a plateau after which further exercise does not increase bone density.

Even low-key physical activity such as walking or gardening will benefit your musculoskeletal system, while also enhancing blood flow that can stimulate the uptake of bone-building nutrients, according to Diane Heislein, MGH orthopedic physical therapist. "No pain, no gain" ain't necessarily so. Depending on the exercise, more vigorous activity may reduce bone loss and fracture to an even greater extent. Yet for some postmenopausal women, vigorous exercise may not be an inviting or realistic goal. Instead, aim to exercise for at least twenty minutes, three days a week; you're under no pressure to run a seven-minute mile.

Unfortunately, few studies to date tell us exactly what type of exercise best benefits bone. Some therapists recommend weight-bearing and resistance-oriented exercises. With weight-bearing exercises, your body weight serves as the load to strengthen muscles and bone, in comparison to resistance training, which makes use of an external load. Weight-bearing exercises include walking and running (hence treadmills and stair climbers), jumping rope, and doing horizontal push-ups. Pedaling a stationary bike is considered a light weight-bearing exercise. Examples of resistance training are weight-bearing aerobics (as opposed to regular aerobics), the lifting of weights, and the pulling and pushing that Nautilus and other equipment provide. The theory is, the more resistance your body encounters, the greater therapeutic benefit for the muscle-bone framework. Some professionals don't recommend resistance training, especially for middle-aged and older individuals, since it can exacerbate back, joint, and muscle problems.

Exercises that put less weight on bones, such as swimming, badminton, or bicycling on flat turf, may not be as effective. "Swimming amounts to nonimpact exercise and it's been clearly shown not to improve bone density," notes Heislein.

Nonetheless, a study done by researchers at the USDA Human Nutrition Research Center on Aging at Tufts University in Boston has signaled that weight lifting can bear impressive bone-related results for certain post-menopausal women. Twice weekly, the formerly sedentary participants used pneumatic resistance machines for forty-five-minute workouts. After a year of training, their hip and back muscles had strengthened by 36 to 76 percent. Their leg and spine bone density increased by 1 percent; their balance improved by 14 percent. In another group of comparably aged women (ages 50 to 70) who remained sedentary, bone density declined as did balance abilities.

For older women, exercise reduces fractures not only by fortifying bone but also by noticeably improving balance, gait, coordination, and response time so that people are less apt to fall and fracture a hip or wrist. If they do fall, they're better able to break their fall, perhaps spraining a wrist but averting a broken hip, an injury that causes complications resulting in death in 15 percent of cases among the elderly. Overall, the strengthening of muscles can simply help the elderly to be more self-sufficient—to do such basic things as get out of a chair or walk to the mailbox.

Researchers such as Dr. Maria A. Fiatarone, chief of the Physiology Laboratory at the USDA Human Nutrition Research Center on Aging at Tufts University in Boston, are helping to spread the word that exercise among the elderly is highly beneficial and safe, provided an individual has no extreme medical problems. Fiatarone and her colleagues have shown that after a few months of high-intensity workouts, frail individuals can regain significant muscle power in their arms, legs, and abdomen, and improve their mobility. One study directed by Fiatarone resulted in a doubling of lower-body muscle strength in elderly women and men after a ten-week exercise program. The average age of the participants was 87.

"Many middle-aged to older women cite time constraints as the main reason they don't exercise. Older women cite the lack of belief that exercise is good for them," says Fiatarone. She maintains that routine exercise can be even better for bone than estrogen replacement. Whereas estrogens serve only to safeguard bone density, exercise can maintain bone density as well as improve muscle mass, muscle strength, and balance, she notes.

At the MGH, Heislein recommends a three-part exercise regimen for postmenopausal women of any age, particularly those whose bones show signs of osteoporosis. The regimen includes a walking program that progressively builds walking time up to twenty to thirty minutes a day; weight-strength exercises that tone the legs and arms; and posture training that strengthens the back and teaches a person the best positions for sitting, bending, and lifting. The specific guidelines of such a regimen are adjusted to meet an individual's needs.

For the sake of your bone, don't run on exercise alone. Remember that calcium and vitamin D are an important part of the picture. Moreover, if your body shows signs of osteoporosis, exercise by itself shouldn't be considered a treatment. A more aggressive approach such as calcitonin or estrogen therapy may be advisable.

10

Nutrition and Exercise: Two Lifelong Prescriptions for Your Heart and Head-to-Toe Health

We Americans are slowly learning how to take better care of ourselves. We are eating more vegetables, fruits, and grain products, and at the same time are cutting back on red meat, total dietary fat, and cigarettes—substances implicated in heart disease and cancer.

But a troubling question remains: When the road to good health is more clearly depicted than ever before, why do so many middle-aged and older Americans have a hard time living healthfully? On average, we're still consuming a reported 34 percent of our total calories from fat, instead of the 20 to 30 percent recommended by nutritionists. And while we should be getting a recommended 60 percent of our total calories from carbohydrates, we're still 10 percent short of that goal.

The recent finding by the National Center for Health

Statistics—that one in three Americans is seriously overweight, as compared to one in four in 1980—is discourag-
ing evidence that many Americans aren't in touch with the
two most important contributors to good health: a sensi-
ble diet and regular exercise.

On average, Americans are consuming 100 to 300 more
calories every day than they used to. For menopausal and
older women, too many extra pounds can have serious
health repercussions. This is especially true because older
women undergo a change in the distribution of body fat.
Fat that once collected around the hips and buttocks—resulting in a "pear" shape—instead starts padding the abdomen—the "apple" shape. This shift in body-fat location
has been shown to be directly linked to a number of health
risks, including heart and circulatory disease, hypertension, gallbladder disease, cancer (primarily endometrial

**Figure 10. Overweight* Trends by Sex and Race, Adults,
Age 20 and Over**

United States, 1960–62 and 1988–91

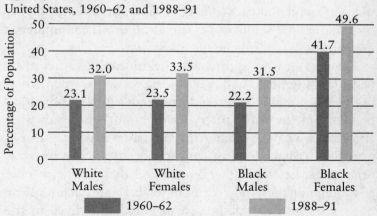

*Approximately 20 percent or more above desired weight.

Source: National Center for Health Statistics; American Heart Association.

cancer), and diabetes. Not surprisingly, excessive weight increases have been shown to closely correlate with increases in death rates.

There's no pat answer to why so many of us cast good sense aside when it comes to health. You know your own reasons best. For many, the trappings of daily life seem to conspire against the maintenance of good health, especially in middle age: jobs that keep us sitting indoors most of the day, restaurants that tempt us with their ribs of beef and creamy desserts, cars that exercise little else but the foot on the accelerator. Moreover, we are surrounded by "marketing and advertising ploys that are aimed at getting us to eat more," notes Sue Cummings, MGH dietitian.

"Menopausal age and older is a very important time to focus on a healthy regimen," emphasizes Cummings. "Too often, many other priorities push nutritional needs to one side." A woman of 50 may feel that making beneficial changes in her diet or physical activity isn't going to make a whole lot of difference. In fact, they can. Since a 50-year-old woman can expect to live, on average, another thirty-two years, how she lives her life at 50 or 60 can influence how she will be faring at age 70 or 80.

Revamping your approach to health can be difficult, especially if ingrained habits block the way. Yet, when crossing the menopause threshold, more and more women are recognizing the value of trying to build better habits. If there's a way of lessening the increased risk for osteoporosis, cardiac disease, cancer, obesity, and numerous other maladies through exercise and diet, why not take advantage of these no-cost nonmedical approaches? Why not try to ensure that the rest of your life is lived to the fullest?

Eating for Health

Most everyone realizes that a proper diet during an individual's growth years is a vital prerequisite for a healthy adulthood. What isn't so widely recognized is that after age 50, eating right is just as important. Many more bodily changes happen during the menopausal and postmenopausal years than most women realize. First, there are all those alterations linked to menopause's depletion of estrogen, progesterone, and androgen—changes affecting muscle, bone, skin, heart, urogenital tissues, body weight, and brain. Concurrently, other aging processes are also altering tissues and systems. With respect to nutrition, vitamins and minerals aren't as easily absorbed as they once were. And since our bodies can't store water-soluble vitamins such as B and C, getting enough of these vitamins becomes all the more important. Add in the fact that many people don't consume all the nutrients their bodies need, and the potential for nutritional problems after age 50 becomes obvious. Because people are living longer than they once did, many nutritionists believe that the nutritional needs of middle-aged and older people are actually greater than what former generations required.

In your menopausal and postmenopausal years, you confront a vexing catch-22: You probably require as many of the basic nutrients as you did in earlier adulthood, or more. Yet because you may be less active and burn off fewer calories, you have lower caloric needs.

Maintaining a sufficient intake of nutrients while consuming fewer calories is a problem for many postmenopausal women. Generally, nutritionists advise that good nutrition is best obtained through what you eat. But dietary supplements may also be necessary, especially since many Americans skimp on the all-important dietary nutrients derived from grains, fruits, and vegetables. A recent government survey revealed that as few as 9 percent of Americans are consuming the recommended daily *minimum* intake of vegetables and fruits. (This amounts to five servings of vegetables and fruits.) As Gladys Block, an epidemiologist at the University of California/Berkeley School of Public Health, told a *New York Times* reporter: "We didn't evolve needing [vitamin supplements]. But the thing is, we did evolve from creatures who got most of their caloric intake from vegetables and fruits, so if we don't eat enough vegetables and fruits, then we may need a supplement factor."

Although supplements can help fill a nutritional gap in diet, it should be remembered that researchers still have a long way to go before they fully understand the value of vitamins and other nutritional supplements. Vitamins were only first isolated during this century. There is still little clear proof of how they "work," and some researchers even suggest that other as-yet-unidentified components in food not found in vitamins may be important for nutrition.

Before you resort to supplements, going back to the basics and eating right is one of the best things you can do for yourself in your menopausal and postmenopausal years. How do you know if you're consuming the appropriate foods and in adequate servings? Let the food pyramid be your guide, and you'll be on course.

The Food Guide Pyramid

Developed by the United States Department of Agriculture in 1993, the food guide pyramid replaced prior guidelines that formerly had emphasized four basic food groups—meat, dairy, fruits and vegetables, and bread. The new pyramid instead focuses on whole grains, fruits, and vegetables. Although the meat and dairy industries weren't especially happy with their foods' lessened status, most nutritionists feel the pyramid's accentuation of whole grains, fruits, and vegetables represents a wiser guide to food selection.

Figure 11. Food Guide Pyramid

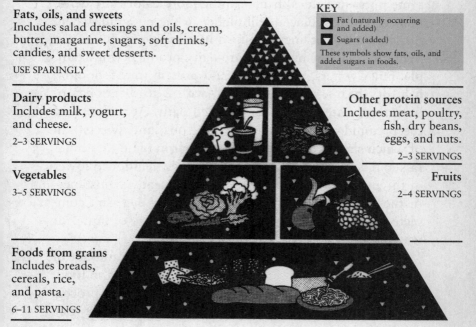

Fats, oils, and sweets
Includes salad dressings and oils, cream, butter, margarine, sugars, soft drinks, candies, and sweet desserts.
USE SPARINGLY

KEY
● Fat (naturally occurring and added)
▼ Sugars (added)
These symbols show fats, oils, and added sugars in foods.

Dairy products
Includes milk, yogurt, and cheese.
2–3 SERVINGS

Other protein sources
Includes meat, poultry, fish, dry beans, eggs, and nuts.
2–3 SERVINGS

Vegetables
3–5 SERVINGS

Fruits
2–4 SERVINGS

Foods from grains
Includes breads, cereals, rice, and pasta.
6–11 SERVINGS

Each of the food groups shown in the pyramid provides some, but not all, of the nutrients you need. Foods in one group can't replace those in another, and no one food group is more important than another. For good health, you need them all.

Source: U.S. Department of Agriculture, and *Via,* March 1994.

The pyramid graphically depicts a balanced intake of vitamins, minerals, carbohydrates, fat, and proteins— which, along with water, constitute life's six essential nutrient categories. As seen in the accompanying illustration, the food pyramid's foundation is devoted to whole-grain foods (bread, cereal, rice, and pasta) with 6 to 11 servings of these recommended each day. On the next level up are vegetables and fruits, with a recommended minimum of 5 servings per day. For total servings, vegetables and fruits are interchangeable. Although both food types have the same nutrient values, fruits can be more calorically dense than vegetables. Placed still higher in the pyramid, where recommended servings diminish in correspondence to the pyramid's narrowing shape, are dairy products (for example, milk, yogurt, and cheese) and protein (meat, poultry, fish, dry beans, eggs, and nuts), with 2 to 3 servings of both these categories recommended daily. At the peak of the pyramid are miscellaneous fats, oils, and sweets—all of which should be used sparingly. Bear in mind that other fats and sugars are also present in foods mentioned lower in the pyramid—the fats found in red meat, for instance, or the sugar derived from fruit. A healthy diet isn't complete without the recommended eight glasses of liquid or water each day.

As the accompanying chart makes clear, the amount of food that counts as a serving can differ from food to food. For instance, one-half cup of pasta, two ounces of process cheese, and one cup of raw spinach each constitutes one serving in its respective food group.

While the food pyramid is a good starting place for getting your nutritional priorities in order, remember that it's designed for all age groups. Because menopausal and older women have different nutritional needs than

Table 5. What Counts as a Serving?

FOOD GROUPS		
Bread, Cereal, Rice, and Pasta		
1 slice of bread	1 oz of ready-to-eat cereal	1/2 cup of cooked cereal, rice, or pasta
Vegetable		
1 cup of raw leafy vegetables	1/2 cup of other vegetables, cooked or chopped, raw	3/4 cup of vegetable juice
Fruit		
1 medium apple, banana, orange	1/2 cup of chopped, cooked, or canned fruit	3/4 cup of fruit juice
Milk, Yogurt, and Cheese		
1 cup of milk or yogurt	1 1/2 oz of natural cheese	2 oz of process cheese
Meat, Poultry, Fish, Dry Beans, Eggs, and Nuts		
2–3 oz of cooked lean meat, poultry, or fish	1/2 cup of cooked dry beans, 1 egg, or 2 Tablespoons of peanut butter count as 1 oz of lean meat	

Source: U.S. Department of Agriculture.

younger women, you'll want to fine-tune the pyramid's offerings, especially for the sake of ensuring a nutrient-rich, low-calorie diet. Here are some suggestions for meeting that goal:

Grains, Fruits, Vegetables

The pyramid's essential message is to focus on whole grains, fruits, and vegetables, and forego excess protein, fats, and sugar. If you are of menopausal age or older, this is especially important. Within these recommended foods lie many valuable complex carbohydrates, vitamins, minerals, protein, and fiber—food factors that researchers believe help protect against cancer and heart disease. (Simple carbohydrates, as opposed to complex carbohydrates, are pure sugar and provide calories but no nutrients. The pyramid makes this distinction, with complex carbohydrates—replete with vitamins, minerals, and fiber—found in foods at the pyramid's base, and simple carbohydrate found at the pyramid's peak.)

Grains, especially whole grains, are rich in complex carbohydrates, which provide the body with an essential source of energy. (Carbohydrates are also found in fruits, vegetables, and dairy products, but not in meats or fats.) Some people mistakenly assume that complex carbohydrates, especially starch, are laden with fat, hence are fattening, but that isn't necessarily true. What often makes carbohydrates fattening is what you add to them—the butter and sour cream topping a baked potato, for instance. Starch, in fact, is the body's most efficient source of energy and gets burned up. Because a high-carbohydrate, low-fat diet is associated with a lower risk of heart disease, diabetes, colon cancer, and other illnesses, postmenopausal women who follow such a diet will be countering health risks developed after menopause.

When buying breads, rice, cereal, pasta, and other grain-derived foods, choose products in which the whole grain has been retained. In comparison, nonwhole, or processed, grains may lack essential nutrients and fiber. When white bread, for example, is processed, parts of the grain kernel have been removed, usually the fibrous bran and the vitamin-rich germ. This helps to ensure a longer shelf life for the product. "Enriched" white bread puts back some of those nutrients that were lost in processing, but not always a full complement of nutrients, according to MGH dietitian Cummings.

"When you purchase a grain product, make sure its label contains the word 'whole,' " advises Cummings. This will mean that the product contains all three grain kernel complements: the germ, the bran, and the endosperm. "Otherwise, if you're buying brown bread, it could be just processed bread that's colored with caramel coloring." If your favorite pizzeria isn't using whole-grain dough, suggest they do so. If the Italian restaurant down the street doesn't yet include whole-grain pastas on its menu, request them.

Along with being less nutritious, fiber-depleted processed grains are not as friendly to the digestive tract as whole grains. Low-fiber diets have been associated with constipation, diverticulitis, hemorrhoids, and colon cancer. Fiber—the nondigestible part of a plant—speeds up the transit of food through the intestine. It can help ward off high total cholesterol, diabetes, and weight gain. A gift for postmenopausal women, fiber has no calories.

The recommended intake for fiber is at least 25 grams a day, or 11.5 grams of fiber for every 1,000 calories consumed. Most people, however, take in less than 10 grams a day, notes Cummings. Although too much fiber consumption can hamper the absorption of calcium, this is less likely to be a problem with fiber derived from food, but may become a problem if a woman is taking too much supplemental bulk fiber.

Along with whole grains, fiber-replete fruits and vegetables provide an excellent way of achieving a low-cal, high-fiber, nutrient-dense diet. "With the exception of avocados, there is no such thing as a high-fat fruit or vegetable," emphasizes Cummings. "Since the food a post-

Table 6. Fiber Facts

Beans and Tofu	Fiber (g)
Health Valley Real Italian Minestrone Soup *(1 c.)* *	11
Pritikin Split Pea Soup *(1 c.)* *	10
Beans *(½ c., cooked)* *	5–8
Lentils *(1 c., cooked)* *	7
Progresso Healthy Classics Lentil Soup *(1 c.)* *	6
Campbell's Black Bean Soup *(1 c.)*[1]	5
Green Giant Harvest Burger *(1)*[2]	5
Progresso Split Pea Soup *(1 c.)* *	5
Mori-Nu Silken Tofu, firm *(3 oz)*	0

Cereals	Fiber (g)
Kellogg's All-Bran with Extra Fiber *(½ c.)*	15
General Mills Fiber One *(½ c.)* *	13
Kellogg's Bran Buds *(⅓ c.)* *	11
Kellogg's All-Bran *(½ c.)* *	10
Nabisco 100% Bran *(⅓ c.)* *	8
Post Raisin Bran *(1 c.)* *	8
Kellogg's Fruitful Bran *(1¼ c.)*	6
Nabisco Shredded Wheat *(2)*	6
Quaker Oat Bran Cereal *(1 c., ckd.)* *	6
Ralston 100% Whole Grain Wheat Chex *(¾ c.)* *	5
Wheatena *(1 c., cooked)*[1]	5
Quaker Quick Oats *(1 c., cooked)* *	4
Quaker 100% Natural Low Fat Granola *(½ c.)* *	4
Total *(¾ c.)* or Wheaties *(1 c.)*	3
Kretschmer Wheat Germ *(1½ Tbs.)*	2
Kellogg's Corn Flakes, Product 19, Rice Krispies, or Special K *(1 c.)*	1

Fruits and Juices	Fiber (g)
Apple *(1)* or Pear *(1)* *	4
Apricots, dried *(⅓ c.)*[1]	4
Blueberries, raw *(1 c.)*	4
Figs, dried *(2)*[1]	4
Apple, without skin *(1)*	3
Banana *(1)* * or Orange *(1)* *	3
Cherries *(1 c.)*[1] or Prunes, dried *(5)*[1]	3
Strawberries *(1 c.)* *	3
Grapefruit *(½)*[1]	2

Table 6 *(continued)*

Grapes *(1½ c.)* or Plums *(2)*	2
Nectarine *(1)*[*] or Peach *(1)*[1]	2
Cantaloupe *(1 c.)*[1]	1
Orange juice *(1 c.)*[1]	1
Watermelon *(2 c.)*	1

GRAINS AND PASTA
(Numbers are for cooked food.) — Fiber (g)

Barley *(1 c.)*[1] or Bulgur *(¾ c.)*[1]	6
Gardenburger *(1)*[*]	5
Aunt Jemima Buckwheat Pancake Mix *(4 4" pancakes)*[2]	4
Brown rice *(⅔ c.)*	3
Couscous, Macaroni[*], or Spaghetti *(1 c.)*	2
White rice *(⅔ c.)*[1]	1

VEGETABLES
(Serving size: ½ cup, cooked.) — Fiber (g)

Green Peas[1]	4
Potato, baked, with skin *(1)*[*]	4
Sweet potato, baked, with skin *(1)*[1]	4
Carrots[1]	3
Asparagus or Broccoli	2
Cabbage[1] or Spinach[1]	2
Carrots, raw, or Corn kernels	2
Cauliflower or Green beans[1]	2
Lettuce, romaine *(1½ c.)*[1]	2
Celery, raw, or Green pepper, raw	1
Lettuce, iceberg *(1½ c.)*[1]	1
Mushrooms, raw *(1 c.)*[1]	1
Tomato, fresh, raw *(½)*[1]	1
Cucumber, sliced, raw	0

BREADS
(Serving size: two slices. Bigger slices help explain why some breads have more fiber—or fat— than others.) — Fiber (g)

Arnold/Brownberry Bran'nola Original or Hearty Wheat[1,2]	6
Oroweat Light 100% Whole Wheat[1]	6
Wonder Light Wheat or 9-Grain[1]	6
Pita, whole wheat *(1)*[1]	5
Roman Meal Light White or Wheat[1]	5

Table 6 *(continued)*

Arnold Oatmeal[1]	4
Roman Meal 100% Whole Wheat[1]	4
Wonder 100% Whole Wheat[1]	4
Tortilla, whole wheat *(1)*	3
Arnold Pumpernickel[1]	2
Pepp. Farm Jewish Seeded Rye[1]	2
Roman Meal Sandwich[1]	2
Pita[1] or Tortilla, white flour *(1)*	1
White[1], French[1], or Vienna[1] bread	1

CRACKERS AND SNACK FOODS *(Serving size: one ounce. The number of crackers, etc., in an ounce is in parentheses.)*	*Fiber (g)*
Wasa Fiber Plus Crispbread *(3)**	9
Wasa Hearty Rye Crispbread *(3)**	7
Wasa Multigrain Crispbread *(3)**	6
Health Valley Fruit Bars *(1)**	4
Nabisco Wheat 'n Bran Triscuits *(7)*[1,2]	4
No-Oil Tortilla Chips *(15–20)*[1]	2–4
Whole Wheat Matzos *(1)*[1]	4
Health Valley Granola Bar *(1)**	3
Nabisco Wheat Thins *(16)*[1,2]	2
Archway Oatmeal Cookies *(1)*[1]	1
Nature Valley Lowfat Chewy Granola Bar *(1)*[1]	1
Quaker Rice Cakes *(1)*[1]	0

* Contains at least 0.6 grams of soluble fiber.
[1] Soluble fiber information not available.
[2] Contains between 4 and 6 grams of fat.
Source: Copyright © 1994 CSPI. Reprinted from *Nutrition Action Healthletter* (1875 Connecticut Ave. N.W., Suite 300, Washington, D.C. 20009-5728. $24.00 for 10 issues.)

menopausal woman consumes has to really count nutritionally, eat as many vegetables as you can and then eat more," she suggests. Myriad studies keep showing that those who consume larger quantities of vegetables are at lower risk for heart disease, cancer, cataracts, and other disorders.

Evidence exists that many fruits and vegetables may be especially beneficial to health because they contain the antioxidants vitamin C and beta-carotene. (Whole grains and nuts contain the antioxidant vitamin E.) Antioxidants are food components that appear to neutralize substances in the body called *oxygen-free radicals,* or *free radicals,* that contribute to cancer, heart disease, and cataracts. Several studies show a correlation between antioxidants and disease protection. However, positive proof of a link between the two is still missing. Some researchers believe that other as-yet-unidentified elements (not necessarily antioxidants) may be blocking free-radical activity. Also, there is controversy over whether the antioxidants in supplements are as effective as those obtained through foods.

A 1996 study indicated that subjects taking beta carotene supplements actually had a higher incidence of death than subjects who didn't take the supplements. Some scientists interpret the results of the study to mean that beta carotene does not have the protective benefits they'd ascribed to it. Other researchers believe that since beta carotene is only one of several related compounds in fruits and vegetables, it may produce benefits only when combined with those compounds as packaged in nature.

Whether or not antioxidants can take credit, a diet rich in fruits and vegetables corresponds with a lower risk for disease, studies show. So you might as well indulge in these foods. Those with antioxidants include many yellow and orange fruits and vegetables: cantaloupe, mango, papaya, pumpkin, sweet potato, and carrot, to name a few.

The phyto-estrogens derived from whole grains, fruits, and vegetables may be another benefit of these three food groups. While research pertaining to phyto-estrogens is preliminary, there's speculation that these mild plant estro-

Table 7. Foods Rich in Antioxidant Vitamins

Vitamin C
U.S. Recommended Daily Allowance
(U.S.R.D.A.): 60 mg

Food	Amount	Mg
Broccoli	1/2 cup	58.2
Brussels sprouts	1/2 cup	35.6
Cantaloupe	1/4 melon	56.4
Cauliflower	1/2 cup	34.3
Clams	1 pint	98.0
Currant, fresh	1/2 cup	101.4
Mango	1	53.7
Green pepper	1	89.3
Hot pepper	1	46.2
Kiwi	1	74.5
Papaya	1	187.8
Orange	1	131.0
Orange juice	6 oz.	155.0
Grapefruit	1/2 fruit	120.0
Grapefruit juice	6 oz.	185.0

Vitamin E
U.S.R.D.A.: 30 mg

Food	Amount	Mg
Dried apricots	1 cup	7.0
Mango	1	2.3
Olive oil	1/2 cup	12.9
Assorted nuts	1 cup	12.9
Pumpkin seeds	1/2 cup	2.5
Fortified cereals	1 cup	27.3
Sweet potato	1	5.8
Wheat germ	3 1/2 oz.	14.1
Sunflower seeds	3 1/2 oz.	44.0
Kale, raw	3 1/2 oz.	8.0

Table 7 *(continued)*

BETA-CAROTENE
There is no U.S.R.D.A. for beta-carotene, but U.S.R.D.A. for
Vitamin A is 5,000 IU.

Food	Amount	IU
Broccoli	1/2 cup	1,082
Carrots, cooked	1/2 cup	19,152
Carrots, raw	1	20,253
Sweet potatoes	1	21,822
Yellow squash	1/2 cup	3,628
Spinach, cooked	1/2 cup	7,371
Spinach, raw	1/2 cup	1,847
Tomato	1	766
Kale, cooked	1/2 cup	2,762
Cantaloupe	1/4 melon	4,304

Excerpted from the March 1993 issue of *The Harvard Heart Letter,* copyright ©
1993, President and Fellows of Harvard College.

gens can help reduce the risk of certain estrogen-related
cancers. Possibly their ability to bind to estrogen receptors
may decrease overexposure to more potent ovarian-made
estrogens. Also, researchers speculate that phyto-estrogens
may cause more estrogen to be absorbed in the intestinal
tract and excreted. Third, phyto-estrogens may fill in for
some of the estrogen lost to menopause, thereby lessening
menopausal symptoms.

Dairy Products

During the menopausal and postmenopausal years, consume low-fat dairy products whenever possible. These can
provide you with as much or more calcium as higher-fat
milk products and help you avoid both unnecessary fat
and calories. You do need some essential fats, but you can
get them by consuming only 1 percent of your diet as fat.

It's worth noting that the food pyramid's recommended 2 to 3 servings/day of dairy products aren't enough to offset the decreased absorption of calcium seen after menopause. Postmenopausally, then, you may need to increase your calcium intake. To do so, consume more low-fat or nonfat milk, yogurt, and cheese, and avoid fat-laden whole-milk cheeses. Try to drink three glasses of low-fat or nonfat milk a day. While a small serving of hard cheese can provide as much calcium as a glass of milk, the accompanying fat calories may be high. Eating more calcium-rich vegetables, such as collard leaves and turnip greens, will help you obtain calcium. A daily calcium supplement will also be necessary for some women. (For a more detailed discussion of dietary calcium and calcium supplements, see Chapter 9.)

Dietary Fat

Your foremost goal over the age of 50 should be to *reduce all fats*. Because postmenopausal women are apt to be less active than in former years, they can't as easily get away with the fried foods, fatty meat, or rich desserts that their younger bodies more easily metabolized. Fat is more readily stored by the body than carbohydrates, contains little nutritional value, may increase total blood cholesterol, and can contribute to cancer, heart disease, high blood pressure, obesity, diabetes, and other ailments. As mentioned before, the body requires just 1 percent of total caloric intake as fat for energy, water storage, and other processes. When you consider that most of us consume 30 percent or more of our daily calories as fat, you can see there's plenty of room for improvement.

All types of fat contain the same number of calories: 9

calories per gram, or more than twice what's found in a gram of carbohydrates. Chemically, fats fall into three basic categories—saturated, monounsaturated, and polyunsaturated—and certain types of fat molecules are more closely associated with coronary artery disease than others. The category to avoid is *saturated* fat, which is mostly found in products derived from animals—red meat, chicken skin, butter, ice cream, cheese, and whole milk, for example. Ice cream and cheese are two of the worst offenders. Saturated fat also exists in some vegetables products, including coconut oil, palm oil, and the cocoa butter that goes into chocolate. Dietitians frequently suggest limiting saturated fat to less than 10 percent of total consumed calories.

As for two other fatty acids—*monounsaturated* and *polyunsaturated* fats—controversy continues over which is nutritionally better or worse. The thinking up until recently has been that monounsaturated fats, which appear mainly in olive, peanut, and canola oils, may be the least harmful. Studies have shown that olive oil and canola oil reduce serum cholesterol without reducing healthy HDL cholesterol. Nonetheless, some essential fats are also derived from *polyunsaturated* fats, which are found in some fish oils and certain vegetable oils (corn, soybean, sunflower, and safflower oils). People consuming too little of certain fatty acids may, in fact, be placing themselves at greater risk for coronary heart disease, maintain researchers.

Until the confusion and unknowns about fatty acids are sorted out, the best advice is to try to resist saturated fats and decrease total dietary fat. Information on the saturated-fat content of a product is now easily found on a product's label. Meanwhile, separating out polyunsaturated from monounsaturated fats isn't always easy, since both can occur in comparable proportions in the same foods. Canola oil, for instance, contains both 59 percent of monounsaturated fat and 30 percent of polyunsaturated, as well as 7 percent saturated fatty acids and other small quantities of fat substances.

Sugars

Like fats, sugar takes up "calorie space" better filled by more nutritious edibles. While moderate amounts of sugar aren't bad for you (aside from contributing to tooth decay), the bountiful calories they so easily bestow are

Table 8. Fatty Acid Content of Oils and Fats*

	Saturated (%)	Monoun-saturated (%)	Polyun-saturated (%)
Beef tallow	50	42	4
Butter	51	23	3
Canola	7	59	30
Chicken fat	30	45	21
Coconut	87	6	2
Corn	13	24	59
Cottonseed	26	18	52
Olive	14	74	8
Palm	49	37	9
Palm kernel	82	11	2
Peanut	17	46	32
Pork lard	39	45	11
Safflower	9	12	75
Sesame	14	40	42
Soybean	14	23	58
Sunflower	10	20	66

* The totals do not add up to 100%, since these oils also contain small amounts of other substances.

Source: USDA Composition of Foods: Fats & Oils.

nearly void of nutrients. In other words, instead of reaching for a Milky Way, you'll be better off downing a sweet peach.

Protein

Like fats and sugar, excess protein all too easily sneaks into the American diet. Although nutritionists usually recommend that protein intake be kept at 10 to 15 percent of overall dietary intake, not infrequently protein accounts for twice that amount. Too much protein often carries with it unnecessary fat intake. If consumed in very excessive amounts, it can also diminish calcium absorption. Generally, six ounces of poultry, fish, meat, or an equivalent of meat protein (from nuts and legumes such as dried peas and beans, for instance) represents the maximum amount of protein that a woman needs each day—a serving portion which is just about the size of the palm of the hand. Since protein is available in vegetables and legumes, soy, whole-grain, and dairy products, it's possible to meet all your dietary protein needs through a diet rich in those foods. Fish protein is also a worthwhile, low-saturated-fat alternative to red meat.

New Food Labels

In 1994 a new comprehensive guide to nutritional information began appearing on food product labels. The new labeling system, developed by the Food and Drug Administration and the U.S. Department of Agriculture's Food Safety and Inspection Service, breaks down the various nutritional components found in one serving of a product based on a 2,000-calorie/day diet. The percentage of the overall daily recommended allowance (now called "Daily Value") that each nutrient per serving represents is also listed. Mandatory components listed include the calories from fat, the total amount of fat and saturated fat (in grams), cholesterol (in milligrams), sodium (in milligrams), total carbohydrate and dietary fiber (in grams), sugar and protein amounts (in grams), and a serving's amount of calcium and vitamins A and C in respect to each nutrient's percentage of the daily value. While the carbohydrates and fats per serving are listed as a percent of total (2,000) calories, the amounts of sodium, cholesterol, and fiber in each serving represent a percent of the maximum amounts recommended each day. Other information that product makers may voluntarily add include a serving's amount of polyunsaturated fat, monounsaturated fat, potassium, and other essential vitamins and minerals.

"The new food labels provide an excellent tool for consumers who want to take charge of their nutritional intake," says Cummings. "For instance, noting the grams of fat and saturated fat can really help a person stay within her individualized recommendation." Cummings emphasizes that it's important to remember that labeling information is based on a 2,000-calorie-a-day diet. "If you're consuming under or over 2,000 calories a day, it may be more useful to focus on total grams rather than percentages."

Weight Tips

As seen in Chapter 4, women have a tendency to gain weight after menopause. Although there is some evidence that weight gain may be tied to hormonal changes, a gradual decline in physical activity as women grow older can also bring on the pounds. Whatever the causes, too many extra pounds can spell trouble, as discussed earlier.

Eating right and focusing on good health are the best approach to weight control, advise many nutritionists. Forced dieting, on the other hand, isn't usually successful, maintains Cummings. "The days of asking a person to go on a 1,200-calorie-a-day diet and giving them a week's worth of menus are over. All too often an all-or-nothing diet doesn't work. In fact, sometimes restricted eating can lead to weight regain. It can make a woman view herself negatively, whereas a less pressured approach to body weight can make her feel more positive about herself and her health," she says. Recent research has shown that as a person loses weight, the body tends to conserve calories, making additional weight-loss that much more difficult.

If you need to lose weight, just sticking to the right foods and fitting more exercise into your schedule, if your health allows for it, can constitute a big step forward. When you follow the food pyramid's guidelines, it's more than likely that pounds will come off gradually. However, while weight loss is desirable for overweight women, reaching an "ideal" body weight isn't always a realistic goal nor a necessary one. As Cummings points out, "It's the first ten to fifteen pounds you lose that are best for your health risk, not the last ten." With those pounds shed, clinical studies have shown, blood sugar and blood cholesterol can drop to desirable levels, which further weight loss doesn't necessarily improve upon.

Cummings and other nutritionists note that current marketing strategies around low-fat products are often misleading. Producers would have you think you can eat more of such products. Yet it's important to remember that low-fat and no-fat foods still contain calories. "Eating a low-fat diet means increasing whole grains, fruits, and vegetables—not eating more low-fat potato chips," advises Cummings.

Of special interest are recent studies showing that when people get into the habit of eating lower-fat foods, over time they can end up preferring a less fatty diet. This changed behavior happens, it seems, because people feel better after eating less fat and because, researchers speculate, a person's taste buds gradually adjust to the taste of lower-fat foods.

That's heartening news: You can eat better and enjoy what you're eating!

Exercising for Health

Diet is only half of the equation for better health. Eating the right foods nourishes the body, but without exercise all you're doing is putting premium fuel in the engine of a car you never take out for a spin.

Although innumerable studies point to exercise's wide-ranging health benefits, fewer than 20 percent of Americans engage in regular exercise after the age of 18. While exercise is a proven preventive of many ills, the medical establishment has been slow in embracing it as such. Regrettably, doctors aren't in the habit of writing out prescriptions for exercise. If they were, exercise might take on the well-deserved reputation of being preventive "medicine" that can produce tangible results.

Mainstream medicine's detachment from exercise often leaves exercise very much of a voluntary pursuit: You're going to have to write out the prescription for yourself. If you can make room for at least twenty minutes of exercise three times a week, you'll be providing yourself with more health advantages than are found in any drug. Exercise has been associated with a lowered risk for high blood pressure, heart attack, diabetes, obesity, numerous intestinal disorders (including ulcers and diverticulosis), diverse cancers, pulmonary disease, and, as seen in the last chapter, bone and muscle deterioration and related fractures. Physical activity can also improve your mental outlook and help you live longer. As long as no health condition bars you from physical activity, pray tell what other "medicine" can so positively impact your health?

> "Six weeks ago I started a walking routine. Five days a week I walk around our neighborhood for about forty-five minutes to an hour. It's had a tremendous releasing effect, just at a time when I badly needed it. My father recently passed away. At my age—50—I'm realizing that it's time to shift priorities and fit in time that can help my health and peace of mind."

Those who begin exercising in their school years appear to reap the greatest benefits from exercise. Nonetheless, the message is increasingly clear these days: It's never too late to start.

Reduced Risk for Heart Disease

Although exercise appears to have less effect on total blood cholesterol levels, research convincingly reveals that routine exercise can substantially increase HDL—the "good cholesterol"—in both men and women. Research into exercise's effects on heart disease in women has been noticeably lacking until recently. However, March 1995 brought a research milestone. Two significant studies reported evidence that exercise indeed yields the same coronary benefits for women as it does men. *Moderate* exercise was found to lower the risk for heart attack by up to 50 percent and the risk for stroke by more than 40 percent.

Moderate exercise (brisk walking or a slow jog) as well as a vigorous workout both appear to improve heart-rate function and general blood circulation, raise HDL, lower blood pressure, and reduce the risk of blood clots. A 60-year-old woman who participates in aerobic workouts may be able to improve her heart-rate function by 25 to 30 percent, one study suggests. A similar-aged woman who walks thirty miles a week may see substantial gains in her HDL cholesterol. Fitness researchers emphasize that sporadic exercise isn't the answer, however. Heart gains depend on a long-term commitment to consistent exercise.

If you have a heart disorder, physical therapy is usually one of the key components in rehabilitation. "One of the first things we do is get them [cardiac patients] exercising as fast and safely as they can," says Miriam Nelson, a physiologist at the Nutrition Research Center on Aging at Tufts. Even for older women who have multiple chronic diseases, specific exercise programs can be an indispensable treatment tool. "Our special goal with such women is to try to make them stronger and more independent," said Nelson.

Reduced Risk for Cancer

One of the least appreciated gifts of exercise is that it appears to play an important role in preventing a broad range of cancers.

For starters, research has shown that regular exercise is correlated with a lower prevalence of colon, bowel, and lung cancer. While physical activity begun early in life is more apt to register greater effects, there are indications that exercise begun in the middle years or later also yields anticancer benefits. Exercise possibly stimulates the production of cancer-inhibiting agents, researchers speculate. It could also help move potential toxins through the colon, lungs, and other organs more rapidly. An important added component is that exercisers, who tend to be on the lean side, are probably consuming lower-fat diets and therefore further protecting themselves against disease.

Studies have found that in later life, former college female athletes experience a lower incidence rate of cancers related to estrogen-sensitive tissue than their sedentary classmates. In the athletes, breast cancer and cancers of the reproductive system (uterine, cervical, ovarian, and vaginal cancer) were significantly less prevalent later in life, as were benign breast and reproductive tumors. Research by Rose E. Frisch—associate professor of population sciences emerita at the Harvard School of Public Health and a pioneer in recognizing exercise's influence on female-specific cancers—and her colleagues has shown that between the ages of 50 and 70, former college athletes often had half the rate of breast and reproductive cancers compared to their nonathlete classmates.

New research indicates that moderate exercise begun years after adolescence but before menopause may still provide protection against breast cancer. Before menopause, the protection may hinge on exercise's ability to influence premenopausal estrogen levels.

"The thinking is that because athletes are leaner, they have less fat cells making estrogen, and therefore less circulating estrogen to affect estrogen-sensitive tissues," says Frisch. "Also, exercisers may be metabolizing natural estrogen to a less potent form." This could result in fewer cells multiplying, hence less risk for a mistake in duplication that could cause cancers to form.

Overall, there's a strong likelihood that exercise continued through menopause, or even initiated after menopause, helps to fend off cancer to some degree. However, research has yet to test this theory. Nonetheless, "The leaner you stay through exercise, the better the whole picture is in terms of cancer," emphasizes Frisch.

Reduced Risk for Lung Disease

Investigations have revealed that if the lungs' airways aren't expanded by occasional deep breathing, they can narrow and become all the more vulnerable to pulmonary diseases that either tighten or block air passages. Exercise can strengthen your respiratory muscles as well as expand your lung capacity. Even if you have certain lung disorders—asthma or chronic constructive lung disease, for instance—your airways can benefit from specific breathing exercises.

Reduced Incidence of Diabetes

Data show that regular exercisers are less susceptible than nonexercisers to adult-onset diabetes. Researchers believe that physical activity allows muscles to remain more responsive to insulin, the hormone that regulates the metabolism of sugar and its entry into muscle cells and other tissues. For individuals with diabetes, regular exercise can minimize the amounts of medication they take and is often considered an integral part of treatment.

Lowered Risk of Severe Gastrointestinal Hemorrhage

A large study of more than 8,200 people 68 years old and older convincingly has shown that even moderate exercise in the later years can ward off the incidence of severe gastrointestinal hemorrhage, a bleeding condition associated with stomach ulcers, diverticulosis, and other illnesses. The National Institute on Aging study found that people who walked or gardened, as well as those who exercised vigorously, benefited from the lowered risk. Researchers theorize that by strengthening blood circulation to the gastrointestinal tract, exercise can help vitalize abdominal tissue. Exercise may also directly ward off the formation of ulcers and other disorders.

Improved Mental Outlook

Anyone who has exercised can't help but notice how the body's quickened tempo has the ability to freshen the mind and the emotions. Exercise has been shown time and again to be an effective tonic for milder forms of depression, a reducer of stress and anxiety, and a booster of energy, self-esteem, and general well-being. The mood-enhancing effects of exercise, it's been shown, can last longer than twenty-four hours. Physical exertion works to clear the mind by reportedly altering serotonin and endorphins, mood-influencing brain chemicals.

"Nothing picks me up mentally like a game of squash. When I'm depressed, I often find it's either because I'm PMS-ish or because I haven't played squash for a week."

Improved Weight Distribution

Not only can regular exercise help you maintain your recommended weight or subtract extra weight, studies have also revealed that as you get older, regular exercise can lessen the chances of fat tissue from collecting around your abdomen. As discussed, this weight distribution pattern, common in many women after menopause, has been associated with an increased risk for heart disease, stroke, and numerous other metabolic disorders.

> "I prefer exercise to estrogen replacement," notes a fit woman in her late seventies. "I religiously walk two miles a day—whether it's sunny or blizzardy. When I read the literature, it's not conclusive that estrogen replacement is a great thing."

If you have no outstanding health problems that could benefit from hormone replacement therapy, it may be far more important to concentrate on exercise and diet in your postmenopausal years than to take hormones on the assumption that they'll magically shield you from illness in later life. There are no substitutes for the benefits derived from diet and physical activity.

End Word

As this book has attempted to show you, menopause is a natural passage and shouldn't be feared. For some women, it will pass by in a blink of the eye, almost unnoticed; for others who stumble onto its transitory symptoms, treatment options exist. As for menopause's associated longer-term effects, such as the increased risk for osteoporosis and heart disease, there too you have numerous choices that can lessen the health-risk consequences and help protect your health in coming years. For all intents and purposes, menopause isn't such a big deal. What *is* a big deal is what it can prepare you for: your health for the remainder of your life. If you notice, learn about, and, if need be, use the nonmedical and medical tools available, the road ahead will be all the smoother. To borrow from Jean-Paul Sartre: "We are responsible for what we are"—and will be.

11

Resources

When it comes to health, there's an increasing trend among women to get below the surface and look for answers—answers about how to maintain good health and how to treat health problems. To that end, the resources mentioned below can be invaluable.

If you want to push your learning curve still higher, innumerable medical journals provide the latest research findings. For the nonscientist, these published reports can be difficult to fathom. Yet most times you'll be surprised by how much you can glean. Since journal subscription costs tend to be high, a well-stocked library is your best source for these publications. Recommended journals for menopausal and older women include:

American Journal of Obstetrics & Gynecology
Fertility and Sterility
Journal of Reproductive Medicine

Journal of the American Medical Association
Journal of Women's Health
Lancet
Maturitas (published by the International Menopause Society)
Menopause: The Journal of the North American Menopause Society
New England Journal of Medicine
Obstetrics & Gynecology

Organizations

American Cancer Society, 1599 Clifton Rd. NE, Atlanta, GA 30329-4251. (800) ACS-2345.

Staffed by nearly two million volunteers and a hard-working group of professionals, this nationwide community-based health organization wages an ongoing fight against cancer through extensive research, public education, and specialized services. Each state has multiple ACS offices, further bridging the gap between you and whatever questions and needs you might have.

American College of Obstetricians and Gynecologists, 409 12th St. SW, Washington, DC 20024-2188. (202) 638-5577.

Members of this nonprofit organization include over 90 percent of American gynecologists and obstetricians. While ACOG mostly serves these professionals, it also publishes many useful pamphlets for the public, such as "Understanding Hysterectomy," "Osteoporosis," "Menopause," and "Hormone Replacement Therapy." Written requests to ACOG should include a self-addressed stamped envelope.

American Heart Association, National Center: 7272 Greenville Ave., Dallas, TX 75231-4596. (800) AHA-USA-1 (800-242-8721).

Supported by over three million volunteers nationwide, the AHA plays a significant role in initiating cardiovascular disease research and in disseminating information about treatment and prevention of heart disease, stroke, and hypertension. Among many free brochures is "Silent Epidemic: The Truth About Women and Heart Disease." Contact the national center or your local affiliate.

American Society for Reproductive Medicine (formerly the American Fertility Society), 1209 Montgomery Highway, Birmingham, AL 35216-2809. (205) 978-5000.

This organization has on hand a wealth of patient information concerning reproductive medicine. Also available upon request is an information booklet on perimenopause and menopause ($1).

Endometriosis Association, 8585 N. 76th Place, Milwaukee, WI 53223. (800) 992-3636, Membership: $25/year

Founded in 1980, the Endometriosis Association is devoted to sharing information with the public and medical community about endometriosis, promoting research, and providing support and help to those afflicted. Members receive a newsletter six times a year. This nonprofit organization can introduce you to a range of helpful educational materials. One of its most popular items is its book *Overcoming Endometriosis: New Help from the Endometriosis Association*—a valuable anthology of articles, fact sheets and research reviews. (Association price: $9.95; bookstore price: $12.95.)

Health Information Network, 4527 Montgomery Drive, Suite E, Santa Rosa, CA (800) 743-6996.

This group specializes in finding print literature on conventional and/or alternative treatment approaches for any medical condition you want to know about. Fees vary according to material requested.

Help for Incontinent People (HIP), P.O. Box 544, Union, SC 29379. (800) BLADDER. Membership: $15/year.

Dedicated to improving the quality of life of people with incontinence, HIP is a leading source of education, advocacy and support. It produces a multitude of pamphlets, videos, tapes, and slide presentations for public use. Members receive a one-year subscription to *The HIP Report* quarterly newsletter and a free *HIP Resource Guide*. This directory of products and organizations assists people in finding the best management solutions.

Hysterectomy Educational Resources and Services Foundation (HERS), 422 Bryn Mawr Ave., Bala Cynwyd, PA 19004. (610) 667-7757.

The HERS Foundation provides information about alternatives to hysterectomy and about coping with the consequences of the surgery. Telephone counseling is free and by appointment. The *HERS Newsletter* is also available. (First issue free; thereafter $20/year for four issues.) For a list of the many articles HERS provides (at $3 each), send HERS a self-addressed stamped envelope.

The Jacobs Institute of Women's Health, 409 12th St. SW, Washington, D.C. 20024-2188. (202) 863-4990. Membership: $40/year.

Founded in 1990 by the American College of Obstetricians and Gynecologists, the Jacobs Institute disseminates information via research, publications, conferences, and workshops for the sake of a better understanding of women's health. Membership includes a subscription to *Women's Health Issues,* a quarterly journal that focuses on pertinent health topics. Members also receive a free copy of the 1995 revised edition of the *Women's Health Data Book: A Profile of Women's Health in the United States.* This volume addresses reproductive health, infectious disease, chronic disease, violence against women, access to the health care system, health concerns among specific groups of women and, in total, a full women's health spectrum. The *Data Book* is available to nonmembers for $28.95, plus shipping and handling.

Melpomene Institute, 1010 University Ave., St. Paul, MN 55104. (612) 642-1951. Membership: $32/year.

Founded in 1982, Melpomene Institute is a research organization devoted to women's health and physical activity. Members receive *The Melpomene Journal,* which carries reports of new research into women's health and general interest articles; discounts on a range of educational products; and the satisfaction of supporting original research on women's physical activity and health.

National Osteoporosis Foundation, 1150 17th St. NW, Suite 500, Washington, DC 20036. (202) 223-2226.

The National Osteoporosis Foundation is the nation's leading resource for patients, health-care professionals, and organizations seeking up-to-date, medically sound information and program materials on the causes, diagnosis, prevention, and treatment of osteoporosis. By contacting the NOF, you can receive a free brochure on osteoporosis and menopause.

National Women's Health Network, 514 10th St. NW, Suite 400, Washington, D.C. 20004. (202) 347-1140. Membership: $25/year.

A nonprofit membership organization, the National Women's Health Network works toward educating health consumers and monitoring legislation that can protect women's health rights. As part of its information services, the network publishes a newsletter *(The Network News)* and numerous well-researched pamphlets. Brochure subjects include "Cervical Cancer/Pap Smears," "Fibroids," "Urinary Tract Infections," "Menopause ERT/HRT," "RU-486," and "Infertility." There's a $5.00 per-packet fee for members and a $7.50 per-packet fee for nonmembers.

North American Menopause Society, c/o University Hospital, 11100 Euclid Ave., Cleveland, OH 44106. (216) 844-3334.

NAMS primarily advances the exchange of research and information among its health-care membership. However, it can furnish you with a list of reading materials, along with a list of recommended gynecologists, support groups, and other health-care providers in your state.

Newsletters and Journals

A Friend Indeed, A Friend Indeed Publications, Inc., Box 1710, Champlain, NY 12919-1710. (514) 843-5730. 10 issues: $30/year.

Published for over a decade, this adeptly written newsletter has been praised for helping to bring menopause "out of the closet." A constant provider of intelligent information, it encompasses the obvious subjects as well as many other underdiscussed topics, such as chemotherapy-induced menopause, menopause and arthritis, and menopausal forgetfulness. Printed letters from readers about their varied experiences enhance the appeal of this monthly review of menopause.

Berkeley Wellness Newsletter, 48 Shattuck Sq., Suite 43, Berkeley, CA 94704. (800) 829-9170. Monthly: $15/year.

Each issue of this eight-page healthletter focuses on how you can prevent disease and promote good health, as opposed to many other healthletters which emphasize diagnosis and treatment. (510) 642-6531/8061.

Environmental Nutrition, 52 Riverside Drive, New York, NY 10024-6599. (800) 829-5384; (212) 362-0424. Monthly: $30/year.

"Open your eyes to what you put in your mouth," urge the compilers of this publication. In a concise fashion, each issue reports on what's safe and healthy to consume, what isn't, and the latest scientific findings that tell the difference.

Harvard Health Letter, Harvard Medical School Health Publications Group, 164 Longwood Ave., Boston, MA 02115. (800) 829-9045. Monthly: $29/year.

This monthly newsletter calls on experts at Harvard Medical School to inform general readers on how to take an active role in staying well and obtaining the best care possible. It interprets complex medical issues and offers thoughtful, in-depth appraisals of the art, science, and economics of modern medicine.

The Harvard Health Publications Group also makes available several special reports: "Postmenopausal Hormone-Replacement Therapy" (which was prepared in consultation with this author in 1993 and updated in 1995), "Sleep Disturbances," "Headache," and "Coronary Artery Disease: Diagnosis and Treatment." ($16 per report)

Harvard Women's Health Watch, 164 Longwood Ave., Boston, MA 02115. (800) 829-5921. Monthly: $24/year.

Begun in the fall of 1993, *Harvard Women's Health Watch* seeks to make sense of the scientific findings surrounding pertinent women's health issues. Each month its eight pages of informative articles invariably cover useful topics for menopausal and older women. Subjects scrutinized in past issues include "Breast Cancer: Environmental Influences," "For Many, Happiness Is a Hysterectomy," "Estrogen and Alzheimer's," and "The Pill Until Menopause?"

Health After 50, P.O. Box 420179, Palm Coast, FL 32142. (904) 446-4675. Monthly: $28/year.

Every article of this Johns Hopkins medical letter is devoted to the health concerns of people age fifty and older. Each issue contains research and advice from professionals at the Johns Hopkins Medical Institutions on menopause, estrogen replacement therapy, or the general health of the postmenopausal woman.

HealthNews, Massachusetts Medical Society, 1440 Main St., Waltham, MA 02154-1649. (800) 848-9155. Seventeen issues: $29/year.

Unlike many wellness journals that focus on prevention and treatment, the newly launched *HealthNews* interprets breaking news in medical research, helping the general public to understand how such advances might affect their health decisions. *HealthNews,* which is made available by the publishers of the *New England Journal of Medicine,* seeks to cut through "confusion and hype" to give its readers "bottom-line recommendations."

Healthy Weight Journal, 402 S. 14th St., Hettinger, ND 58639. (800) 663-0023. Bimonthly: $59/year. Student rate: $27/year.

Healthy Weight Journal provides a critical link between research and recommendations for maintaining your weight. It covers the causes behind weight gain and loss, the prevention of weight problems, weight-related disease risks, and the treatment of obesity and eating disorders. The journal's compilers have also published two special reports: "Health Risks of Obesity" contains current statistics on both the risks of obesity and its treatment (192 pages/ $29.95). "Health Risks of Weight Loss" establishes that many current weight loss treatment methods aren't good for your health and reviews the "nondiet" movement (160 pages/ $19.95).

Hot Flash: Newsletter for Midlife and Older Women, Box 816, Stony Brook, NY 11790-0609. Quarterly: $25/year.

Hot Flash, published by the National Action Forum for Midlife and Older Women, presents up-to-date information about the physical, emotional, and social concerns of women.

Mayo Clinic Health Letter, Mayo Foundation for Medical Education and Research, 200 First St. SW, Rochester, MN 55905. (800) 333-9037. Monthly: $24/year.

In an easy-to-understand style, this newsletter offers practical health information on timely topics, enhanced by full-color medical illustrations and photographs.

Menopause Management, Carrington Communications, Inc., P.O. Box 658, Flanders, NJ 07836. (201) 584-3040. Bimonthly: $65/year.

Endorsed by the North American Menopause Society, this journal provides practical clinical guidelines—not research findings—regarding how to manage peri- and postmenopausal health. Although written primarily for health-care professionals, you'll find it extremely readable and packed with excellent advice and opinions by prominent authorities.

Menopause News, 2074 Union St., San Francisco, CA 94123. (415) 567-2368. Bimonthly: $23/year.

Menopause News looks at significant research findings and trends as well as the people who contribute to an understanding of menopause. It covers everything from research connected to the Women's Health Initiative to the latest developments in menopause clinics and hormone regimes. A first-person feature article and a "Letters" section add helpful insight.

MidLife Woman, MidLife Women's Network, 5129 Logan Ave. S., Minneapolis, MN 55419-1019. (612) 925-0020/(800) 886-4354. Bimonthly: $25/year.

MidLife Woman offers detailed information about health and menopause. Well written and carefully researched, each issue of *MidLife Woman* presents an in-depth review of one specific topic as well as news updates concerning women's health and book reviews. Past issues have focused on hysterectomy, new research into menopause, and the emotions of midlife. The MidLife

Women's Network also offers written programs on menopause with slides for individual or group use.

Nutrition Action Healthletter, Center for Science in the Public Interest, Suite 300, 1875 Connecticut Ave. NW, Washington, DC 20009-5728. (202) 332-9110 or (800) 237-4874. 10 issues: $24.

It's no wonder that *Nutrition Action Healthletter* has the largest circulation of any newsletter of its kind in the country. Full of full-color photos, drawings, graphs, and charts, its sixteen pages yield absorbing information that pulls in the eye as well as the mind. The contents cover personal health, advocacy activities, and important nutrition research. Will pasta make you fat? What nutritional values await you in a Mexican, Chinese, or French restaurant? How should food be stored and kept safe at home? This healthletter cuts straight to the bone.

Tufts University Diet and Nutrition Letter (newsletter), 203 Harrison Ave., Boston, MA 02111. (617) 482-3530 or (800) 274-7581. Monthly: $20/year.

This newsletter gives readers the tools to manage a balanced diet. Monthly features include nutritional comparisons of various foods and beverages; questions and answers; book reviews; and in-depth reports on such topics as exercising in older age, diagnosing lactose intolerance, and mail-order houses that provide the best cooking ingredients.

The University of Texas Lifetime Health Letter, The University of Texas-Houston Health Science Center, 7000 Fannin, Houston, TX 77030. Customer Service: (800) 829-9177. Monthly: $24/year.

Devoted to useful news concerning health, fitness, and nutrition, this monthly newsletter is specially slanted toward mid-aged and older readers and how they can live longer and healthier lives.

VIA: A Guide Through Menopause and Beyond, Carrington Communications, P.O. Box 658, Flanders, NJ 07836. (201) 584-3040. Quarterly: $19.97/year.

VIA encourages women to expand their knowledge of health-care issues, particularly concerning peri- and post-menopause. Nationally known contributing editors provide regular columns addressing key topics, such as nutrition, fitness, psychology, and sexuality. Features cover pressing medical concerns and dispel myths.

Women's Health Advocate, Amicus Publishing, 3918 Prosperity Ave., Fairfax, VA 22031. Subscriptions: (800) 829-5876. Monthly: $24/year.

Said one reader, "Reading [this newsletter] is like sitting around with a group of women doctors and friends, taking part in a conversation about the best ways of protecting our health and wellness." With an editorial review board made up of professional women health-care providers, the assorted health news and advice found here is solidly woman-to-woman.

Books

Breast Cancer? Breast Health! The Wise Woman Way by Susun Weed. Ash Tree Publishing, P.O. Box 64, Woodstock, NY 12498. Phone/Fax: (914) 246-8081; 356 pages.

A new release, this guide to natural treatments contains suggestions of herbs, foods, energy techniques, and home remedies that can promote breast health as well as supplement breast surgery, radiation and chemotherapy.

Menopausal Years: The Wise Woman Way by Susun S. Weed. Ash Tree Publishing, P.O. Box 64, Woodstock, NY 12498. Phone/Fax: (914) 246-8081. Paper: 228 pages.

Sharing advice passed down through generations, herbalist Susun Weed provides information into a range of natural remedies for peri- and postmenopausal symptoms and conditions. In particular, specific herbs are reviewed for their treatment effects.

Menopause, Naturally: Preparing for the Second Half of Life by Sadja Greenwood, M.D. Volcano Press, P.O. Box 270, Volcano, CA 95689-0270. (800) 879-9636.

Gloria Steinem has referred to *Menopause, Naturally* as a "commonsense guide for this rite of passage." In this newly released fourth edition, Dr. Greenwood has incorporated new material on the causes, prevention, and treatment of osteoporosis, new knowledge about the value of soybeans in the diet, and an up-to-date discussion of hormone replacement therapy.

The New Ourselves, Growing Older: Women Aging with Knowledge and Power by Paula B. Doress-Worters and Diana Laskin Siegal; Simon & Schuster, 1994. Paper: 531 pages.

First released in 1987 in cooperation with the Boston Women's Health Book Collective, *Ourselves, Growing Older* won many readers with its positive approach and helpful guidance. This new edition, updated in 1994, similarly embraces a wide range of subjects, including menopause, body image, sexuality, career, retirement, and housing. As Tish Sommers notes in her foreword, "Since we cannot beat aging, we had better learn how to join in."

The Osteoporosis Handbook: Every Woman's Guide to Prevention and Treatment by Sydney Lou Bonnick, M.D., Taylor Publishing Co., 1550 West Mockingbird Lane, Dallas, TX 75235. (214) 637-2800/(800) 275-8188. Paper: 192 pages.

The North American Menopause Society cites this book as "a comprehensive, factual, concise, and readable review of the whole subject" of osteoporosis. It includes information about diagnosis, diet, supplements, and exercise and responds to the fifty most-asked questions about bone loss.

Without Estrogen: Natural Remedies for Menopause and Beyond by Dee Ito, Crown Trade Paperbacks. Paper: 272 pages.

Without Estrogen is for women who can't or choose not to take estrogen and are seeking alternative therapies to alleviate menopausal symptoms and strengthen their health. A group of alternative practitioners offers recommendations. Also heard from are eleven women who describe their programs of herbs, vitamins, exercise, and other therapies, giving their assessments of each therapy's successes and failures. This newly released paperback version makes this advice all the more affordable.

Video and Audiotapes

Menopause Metamorphosis (video). Ash Tree Publishing, PO Box 64, Woodstock, NY 12498. Phone/Fax: (914) 246-8081. $29.95; 55 minutes.

This video features herbalist and author Susun Weed and a small group of women ages 38 to 63 talking candidly about perimenopause, menopause, and simple home remedies for uncomfortable menopausal symptoms.

Those Middle Years (audio tape set), ColorSong Productions, Box 120321, St. Paul, MN 55112. (800) 352-6567. $29.95; 3 hours.

This tape set, hosted by psychologist and family therapist Janice Winchester-Nadeau, Ph.D., openly and candidly discusses a woman's and man's journey through the passage of midlife. Frank discussions of menopause, intimacy and sexuality, loss and grief, and other issues of this passage provide the listener with helpful insights. The tapes are replete with poetry as well as original music by singer-songwriter Ken Medema.

Index

About the Author

D<small>R</small>. I<small>SAAC</small> S<small>CHIFF</small> is Chief of Vincent Memorial Obstetrics and Gynecology Service at Massachusetts General Hospital and Joe Vincent Meigs Professor of Gynecology at Harvard Medical School. In 1976 he initiated one of the first menopause clinics in North America. A former president of the North American Menopause Society, he is currently editor-in-chief of the journal *Menopause*. His major interest is the clinical care of his patients.

A<small>NN</small> B. P<small>ARSON</small>, a freelance journalist, writes on subjects pertaining to health, science, the environment, and golf. She also teaches science journalism at Boston University.